Understanding Patients

Paul Morrison
BA PhD RMN RGN PGCE CPsychol AFBPsS
Senior Lecturer, School of Nursing Studies
University of Wales College of Medicine,
Cardiff, UK

Baillière Tindall
London • Philadelphia • Toronto • Sydney • Tokyo

Baillière Tindall   24–28 Oval Road
W. B. Saunders   London NW1 7DX

The Curtis Center
Independence Square West
Philadelphia, PA 19106–3399, USA

Harcourt Brace & Company
55 Horner Avenue
Toronto, Ontario, M8Z 4X6, Canada

Harcourt Brace & Company, Australia
30–52 Smidmore Street
Marrickville
NSW 2204, Australia

Harcourt Brace & Company, Japan
Ichibancho Central Building
22–1 Ichibancho
Chiyoda-ku, Tokyo 102, Japan

A catalogue record for this book is available from the British Library

ISBN 0–7020–1718–3

Typeset by Fakenham Photosetting Limited, Fakenham, Norfolk
Printed and bound in Great Britain by Mackays of Chatham, plc

Contents

Foreword

There are those in influential positions, within and without the NHS, who would wish to roll back the years and reduce nursing again to a task focused way of working. They would substitute getting the jobs done for holistic care and replace nursing education with an old style apprenticeship. It is therefore essential for the future of the nursing profession that we understand and value the importance of treating the patient as a whole person rather than a collection of tasks. Insight into the patient's experience of the health care system is therefore critical to the implementation of a holistic nursing philosophy. This is what Paul Morrison offers us in this thought-provoking book.

Research studies which have tried to discover the degree of patient satisfaction with care received have failed to achieve any degree of discrimination between good and bad care. There are many reasons for this failure which flow partly from the patient's perception of care and partly from the methodology used. This book tackles this problem from a very different angle and sheds far more light on the problems as a result.

This text deserts the traditional empirical paradigm of scientific enquiry which in the past has relied upon 'tick box' methods to try and discover how patients felt about their care. In place of this approach we find a very different qualitative style of research, drawing upon patients' own accounts, to paint a rich picture of what it feels like to be a patient. This refreshing break with conventional research methods allows the reader to gain genuine insights into patient perceptions and also demonstrates the advantages to be gained from using alternative research strategies. It does nursing research a great favour in the process.

The key to successfully implementing a holistic nursing philosophy lies in understanding the patient's point of view. This text will help all nurses achieve that perspective while demonstrating the value of qualitative research. These are two key battles that have to be won in securing the future of nursing as an independent profession in its own right.

Mike Walsh PhD
Head of Department,
Nursing and Midwifery,
St Martin's College,
Lancaster, UK

Acknowledgements

Several people have helped to shape my thoughts and ideas over the last 9 years. Professor Peter Ashworth has been very influential. He supervised my PhD study and guided me through all the difficult stages that a research degree usually entails. He patiently supported me as I struggled to come to terms with some of the most important principles of phenomenological psychology. Philip Burnard and Jim Richardson have been very supportive colleagues and good friends.

The patients who took part in the study also taught me a great deal. They reminded me of the great responsibility that professional carers have and of the need to be an 'ordinary' person who happens to be a nurse or other professional helper.

Chapter 1
Introduction

This book is aimed primarily at students and practitioners in nursing and at other professional helpers who have, as the focus of their work, relationships with clients, patients and their families. Although the official rhetoric of many professional helping agencies suggests that the care received by patients and clients in hospital and community settings is 'individualized' and 'person-centred', in reality it is not.

There are of course many possible reasons for why this is so. One of the main reasons for this discrepancy is the professionals' general lack of understanding of the people they care for. Members of the nursing profession and other helping professions have been ill-served by the forms of human science research that are currently dominant, many of which have failed to provide a clear and full understanding of patients and their experiences.

This book attempts to put forward a descriptive but research-based account of the lifeworld of the patient. It cannot reflect the concerns of all patients receiving professional care but it does offer professional carers a framework for developing an understanding of the individual people they care for. It will help practitioners to begin to comprehend the patients' experiences of being cared for in a hospital context, and in so doing it will offer the professional nurse the opportunity to think carefully about the concept of 'individualized' nursing care. Diploma and Degree nursing students, whatever branch of nursing they are undertaking (child, adult, mental health or care of the person with learning difficulties), will find something of interest in this book.

Nurses engaged in types of qualitative research that require a detailed insight into the world of another person, will read the following chapters with interest. The rich data collected during the interviews with patients produced findings that reflected the issues and concerns of ordinary patients in hospital. They will, however, need to follow-up some of the references and further readings for more in-depth methodological debates, discussions and practical guidelines on how to execute qualitative interviews.

While there are many books about nurses and nursing practice that consider the patient and his or her needs, there are no books of this nature available that offer the combination of a psychological research base and an in-depth understanding of the patients' world. It is this combination of factors that has enormous potential for improving the quality of professional nursing practice.

Features of the book

This book is about patients' experiences of the care received in hospital.

- It is based partially on research completed for a PhD degree. In that study the personal experiences of nurses and hospital patients were explored and described. The nurses who took part in the study were asked to relate their 'experiences of caring for patients' in a professional setting. The patients were asked about their experiences of 'being cared for'. Only the patients' perspective is examined here. The emphasis on the patient perspective is deliberate and appropriate. In nursing research the emphasis has fallen on the nurses' world and a more balanced perspective needs to be achieved. Without patients there would be no need for nurses. This book will help to emphasize the patients' perspective.

- The personal accounts and experiences described are of patients in a 'general' hospital but that general hospital perspective is not particularly limiting. The experiences related by patients during research interviews evoked many common features that mental health nurses, children's nurses and other healthcare workers will readily identify.
- The approach used in the research is not widely used, although it is rapidly gaining in popularity and particularly so in nursing research (see for example Watson, 1985; Benner and Wrubel, 1989; Gullickson, 1993). The particular approach used emphasized an 'existential' understanding of the experiences of hospitalized patients. It highlighted a descriptive account of the patients' 'lifeworld'—the world that they experience and live.
- The words and phrases that the patients themselves used to describe their experiences have been used throughout the text. These personal accounts have been written as small 'snapshots' and from time to time some verbatim quotations from the interview transcripts have been added to give the reader a flavour of the interviews and the way patients conversed during these interviews.
- One of the aims of writing this book was to encourage nurses to *think* more about their work and to help them *understand* more fully those people in care. The book has been set out from the perspective that *patients are people first* and patients later. All healthcare workers could be encouraged to approach their work from this perspective. Such an approach could lead to improvements in the care received by patients, but the challenge of providing 'holistic' or 'individualized' care to patients is great. Higher standards of care can be achieved if nurses

develop approaches to patients that 'involve' patients more fully in their care (Ashworth *et al.*, 1992).

- Nurses must be able to provide competent nursing care to those they are paid to care for. This means that they must be proficient in the 'basic' and 'technical' facets of care as well as the 'human' facet of care. Together these facets comprise a unified approach to nursing people. Whatever the branch or specialty of nursing, all nurses need particular skills and attitudes to help them to do the job well. The potential for working in a more 'patient-centred' way can be achieved by reading about the experiences of patients who have received care and using this information for reflecting on nursing work.

- The description of the patients' experiences of receiving care in hospital reinforced many of the findings that have already been described in the research literature. The fact that these concerns reappeared in this study may be taken as further evidence of the need for nurses to manage these 'problem areas' more effectively. In addition, the emotional aspects of the patients' experiences was striking and moving. This emotional constituent of the patients' experiences highlighted the need for different groups of professional carers to deal more effectively with the emotional aspects of caring for patients.

- Converting one aspect of a research study into a more accessible and more widely readable form was a difficult task. The aim has been to emphasize the patients' experiences of care in a hospital setting by describing the experiences of a small group of patients. My purpose was to encourage readers to think carefully about the patients in their care and about their own style of providing care. A series of revisions was therefore needed to produce a less 'academic' and more 'friendly' book that would serve to remind nurses and other carers about the world experienced by patients. The level of referencing has been kept to a minimum and each chapter has a specific list of further reading. The reader is encouraged to explore particular issues in greater depth in those journals and books.

An outline of the book

In Chapter 2 some of the basic principles of phenomenological psychology have been sketched briefly. In particular, the 'existential' perspective has been described and the concept of the 'lifeworld' emphasized. This approach underpinned the research that forms the basis of the later chapters of the book. It was used to interview nurses and patients. The phenomenological approach has rapidly gained acceptance amongst researchers in healthcare settings, especially where investigators have tried to examine the individual way in which people respond to treatment or cope with chronic illness and disease (Morse, 1989).

The principles identified in this chapter were used to guide the setting up of interviews with patients. They influenced the type of questions that were asked and the way in which questions were asked. These principles affected the way in which the interview data were analysed and interpreted. Hopefully, the straightforward style of writing and the insights into patients' experiences that are illustrated throughout the remainder of the text will convey how this theoretical foundation may be transformed in an 'applied' way to nursing work and caring in practice. It may be helpful to read Chapter 2 a couple of times.

Some of the traditional ways of thinking about the patients' situation in hospital have been explored briefly in Chapter 3. The theory of learned helplessness (Seligman, 1992) has proved to be a useful framework for considering patients in hospital or other institutions. This is especially so when considering patients receiving long-term care in institutional settings—the elderly, mentally infirm, people with learning disabilities—or chronically disabled individuals. The theory helps to promote an understanding of the complex social setting in which professional care is given. It also helps us to understand how patients and nurses think, feel and behave.

Another psychological theory referred to in Chapter 3 deals with interpersonal perception. Attribution theory helps us to identify some of the subtle ways in which nurses and patients perceive each other. The role of attributions in labelling patients as 'good' or 'bad' is examined. The process of making attributions can influence the 'sick role' that many patients adhere to in hospital.

In Chapter 4 one of the four major themes found to characterize patients' experiences of receiving care is described in detail and discussed. The patients were cared for at a time of 'crushing vulnerability'. This important theme is explored and many subtle differences in patient perceptions were found to unfold during a detailed analysis of this theme. The feelings of 'depersonalization' or of being made to feel like an 'object' rather than a person were particularly important facets of vulnerability for these patients.

Vulnerable patients have to adapt to the strange hospital environment, to illness and to the role of an ill person. The modes of self-presentation that were used by the patients in this study have been described in Chapter 5. Many different types of self-presentation were identified and described, of which several seemed to be child-like, unhelpful and unadaptive. Some patients became 'sheepishly obedient', were 'unusually friendly and cheerful' or showed 'deference and gratitude for the carers'. These modes of self-presentation emerged from the patients' vulnerable and powerless position in the social situation that characterizes the organizational structures found in hospital. Although these modes of self-presentation may help patients to adapt and cope with illness and hospital in the short term, they are unlikely to lead patients to assume greater responsibility for their own health care in the long term. This process of adaptation may inadvertently promote dependence on professional assistance from nurses, doctors and other healthcare workers.

In Chapter 6, the patients' evaluations of the 'hotel services' are outlined. There was generally a high level of satisfaction with the standards of care they observed and experienced. Patients focused their attention on small details that may seem unimportant to the nurse. However, these unimportant aspects of hospital life may send a message to patients. The hotel services may be 'symbolic': a high standard of hotel services tells patients they are worthy of care and attention, while a poor standard tells them the opposite.

Although there was generally a high level of satisfaction with services provided, some patients highlighted important points that the professional nurse ought to consider carefully. Patients had very little contact with the staff and almost no contact with the trained and most experienced nurses on the wards. The students were singled out for particular praise— having a helpful attitude and always being available for patients meant a great deal to those patients. Students took time to talk to patients. In general, patients seemed unwilling to be too critical of the 'system'. Perhaps they were feared that making even a minor criticism of the staff would result in less professional attention and care. They feared being ignored by the staff. Finally, the unequal status of the patient and nurse was also evident in this theme.

The 'personal concerns' of the patient are dealt with in Chapter 7. Nurses often claim to make assessments of patients that encompass all the important elements in that person's life (physical, psychological and social spheres), and to generate care plans around these—total patient care, holistic or individual care. This was certainly not so with the patients who took part in this study. During the interviews patients revealed details about their lives outside hospital that surely influenced their reactions as patients. The staff were not aware of these details.

The 'treatment' was uppermost in the minds of some, while the 'frustration' at being in hospital was very disruptive in another patient's life. One patient had had bad experiences with her family doctor and another had not really come to terms with her mother's recent death. These sorts of issues were disclosed openly to an unfamiliar researcher during interviews. The nurses on the ward ought to have known about these things. They could have helped the patients to deal with the anxiety that these personal concerns must have produced. However, given that the contact between trained nurses and patients was limited, just as it appears to be so in many other studies of hospitalized patients, it was unlikely that opportunities for open communication existed. This is an issue that nurses must address. The findings described in Chapters 4–7 raise many important questions for practising nurses.

In Chapter 8 a more detached perspective has been adopted and some of the critical issues that encroach on the 'professional caring relationship' have been reviewed. The ideas of power, mutuality and commitment are discussed. The importance of the 'physical' care has been emphasized because it helps the nurse to build a 'bridge' for providing psychological care for patients. Paradoxically, the more training and experience a nurse acquires, the less likely she or he is to use that knowledge and experience with patients directly. This raises important issues for training and for the management of nursing services. Several important dilemmas facing all professional carers such as nurses, doctors, social workers and clinical psychologists, have also been outlined briefly in this chapter.

In the final chapter of the book some of the potential areas where the phenomenological perspective could be used to promote a greater understanding of patients and clients are outlined. To achieve the goal of 'really understanding patients' will entail change at the individual and organizational level. It will involve personal commitment, patience and planning. Some training materials are already available but a great deal of work still needs to be done. Some suggestions for promoting change are offered.

Personal commitment

In several chapters a small section on 'what can be done to improve the situation' has been included to encourage people to think carefully about their own work and the work of the unit or clinic where they are currently placed. Introducing change on a large scale in organizations is difficult and demanding and usually takes a long time. However, with a 'personal commitment' to develop and change, individual nurses can do a great deal and positively influence those they work with. Individuals should not underestimate their ability to change things, especially if they work within a small group of people. People who are willing to take responsibility and work hard can make things happen. Adopting the approach outlined here will entail changing *your* attitudes.

The 'patient'

As I re-read the draft chapters of this book I noted how entrenched the term 'patient' is in my own vocabulary. The word 'patient' frequently elicits a range of related constructs— powerless, conforming, bad and good, obedient, vulnerable and so on. It emphasizes the difference in status between professional carers and those who are ill. I considered changing the word patient but was unhappy with the alternatives. They all seemed clumsy and wordy—the ill person, the person in hospital, the sick individual and so on. While acknowledging the disadvantages of using the word 'patient' from the patient's perspective, it must be acknowledged that the word is used widely in practice and will for the foreseeable future remain a common term. On those grounds I decided to use the word 'patient' throughout. All the patients' names used throughout the book are false names.

Chapter 2
Exploring personal experience

If you really want to help somebody, first of all you must find him where he is and start there. This is the secret of caring. If you cannot do that, it is only an illusion, if you think you can help another human being. Helping somebody implies you are understanding more than he does, but first of all you must understand what he understands. If you cannot do that, your understanding will be of no avail. All true caring starts with humiliation. The helper must be humble in his attitude towards the person he wants to help. He must understand that helping is not dominating, but serving. Caring implies patience as well as acceptance of not being right and of not understanding what the other person understands (Kierkegaard, 1859, cited in Davis and Fallowfield, 1991).

Introduction

The nursing profession is changing rapidly. Within a few short years, the education of nurses has become part of the system of higher education in different countries and many experienced nurses are now returning to the educational arena to obtain basic and higher degrees. Practitioners and educators have come to recognize the importance of a research base for practice and a significant number of nurses are actively engaged in research projects. A growing number of nurses are undertaking research degrees.

The clinical role of the nurse has become more demanding and challenging. The management of hospitals and community services has changed and continues to change, and these changes have affected the way nurses work. There is an increased awareness of the need to provide high quality care for individual patients and their families. Nurses and other healthcare workers have assumed greater responsibility for ensuring that patients' needs are met. The growth of consumerism in the health service arena means that patients' expectations of the service are more explicit.

The developments in nursing have led to an increased awareness of the importance of psychology and psychological care in nursing practice. Students, practitioners and researchers have become more attentive to the psychological needs of the patient, but there is still a long way to go. One major facet of psychological care is the need to *understand the patient*. This book deals with the process of understanding patients using the phenomenological school of psychology.

In this chapter some of the theoretical principles that form the basis of phenomenological psychology are explored. These are important stepping stones for developing a clear picture of how this theoretical approach may be used to guide human research. A primary objective of this approach is to develop an understanding of personal experience as it is 'lived'. This perspective underpinned a study into the experiences of nurses and patients, but only the patients' experiences have been described in the following chapters.

This phenomenological approach has increasingly found favour with a growing number of psychologists and other healthcare researchers, including nurses. More importantly, the approach can be used to help practitioners to develop skills in *understanding* their patients and clients more fully. This understanding could in turn lead to changes in policy and practice and ultimately to improvements in the quality of care received by patients.

Selecting a psychological approach

Psychology can be defined broadly as the study of human experience and behaviour. The scope of study is huge and there are many different approaches to studies in psychology (see for example Atkinson *et al.*, 1990; Gleitman, 1992). Some psychologists prefer to focus on the biological bases of behaviour. They study the person at a 'cellular' level and try to establish, for example, how the brain and nervous system works and how it influences behaviour and emotions. Others focus on particular psychological processes such as 'learning', 'thinking' or 'memory'.

At the other extreme there are some psychologists who emphasize the 'social' aspects of human activity and focus their studies on the ways in which people interact in pairs or in small groups. Any psychological approach to the study of human experience must also be rigorous and testable. In other words it must be seen to be an accurate representation of how people experience life.

One thing is clear: psychologists are interested in people. Nurses are people who care for sick people in a specific way and in a particular context. Nurses therefore need to know about the work that psychologists do and to learn how a psychological approach can help them to look after patients in more informed and effective ways. While there are many different approaches in psychology that could be useful to nursing students, the particular approach described here offers enormous potential when applied to the field of nursing. The approach discussed in the remainder of this chapter has been described as phenomenological psychology (Giorgi, 1970).

Although the foundation for this type of psychology may be traced to a much earlier time, the approach has only become a more widely accepted part of psychological science in the last 25 years. Spiegelberg (1982) has provided an extensive history of the 'phenomenological movement', but it is not the easiest place to start reading about phenomenological psychology. The approach emerged because a number of psychologists who were interested in humans rather than animals, expressed 'strong feelings of dissatisfaction with psychology's standard means of coping with the phenomena of human experience' (Giorgi *et al.*, 1971, p. xi). The driving force behind this approach was the need to describe reality within a *social and human context*:

> More specifically, the issue is to find means of studying perception, learning, etc. while at the same time being mindful of the human-ness of the subject and the social aspects of the situation. Thus, there is a deliberate attempt to break away from basically physicalistic expressions of the world and to move toward more experiential descriptions (Giorgi *et al.*, 1971, p. xii).

The existential–phenomenological approach

The phenomenological approach is both a philosophy and a method of analysis for qualitative research data. In the research context, the phenomenological approach facilitates the study of consciousness and personal experience. The researcher is required to try and put aside (or bracket) his or her own assumptions and prejudices to ensure that the viewpoint of the *person being studied* is reported clearly:

> The phenomenologist views human behaviour, what people say and do, as a product of how people define their world. The task of the phenomenologist. . .is to capture this process of interpretation. . .the phenomenologist attempts to see things from other people's point of view (Taylor and Bogdan, 1984, pp. 8–9).

A method to enable researchers to achieve these goals was provided by Edmund Husserl (1972), the founder of the philosophy of phenomenology. Husserl emphasized the need to study human consciousness and experience in a methodologically rigorous way by focusing on the 'experienced' world or lifeworld. Here, the researcher attempts to study everyday experience as it is *lived* and to develop deeper insights into the lived world of human experience. The researcher does not seek validation for his or her own theories, but tries instead to minimize the effect of any pre-conceived ideas or personal bias. Spinelli (1989) outlined three major components of Husserl's phenomenological method as follows:

- There is an emphasis on the need to *bracket* or set aside our expectations and assumptions so that we can be open to our current experiences and accurately interpret them.
- There is a need to *describe* the conscious experience fully without attempting to explain it to arrive at the *essence* of that experience.
- It is assumed that all aspects of the description are treated as equal, and no attempt is made to organize them hierarchically.

The particular approach that Husserl (1972) advocated was primarily concerned with the description of *essences* (what makes something what it is) in human consciousness and experience.

A closely related but different approach was developed by the German philosopher Martin Heidegger (1962). The emphasis within Heidegger's approach was placed on human *existence* (Heidegger, 1962; Macquarrie, 1973). This accent elevated the question of existence to a position of prime importance in phenomenology and led to the development of the existential perspective in phenomenological psychology. The existential position has three essential concerns. These have been summarized by Stevenson (1987) briefly as follows:

The first is with the *individual* human being, rather than with general theories about him. Such theories, it is thought, leave out what is most important about each individual—his uniqueness. Secondly, there is a concern with the *meaning* or purpose of human lives, rather than with scientific or metaphysical truths about the universe. So inner or subjective experience is typically regarded as more important than 'objective' truth. Thirdly, the concern is with the *freedom* of individuals as their most important and distinctively human property. So existentialists believe in the ability of every person to choose for himself his attitudes, purposes, values, and way of life. And they are concerned not just to maintain this as a truth but to persuade everyone to act on it. For in their view the only 'authentic' and genuine way of life is that freely chosen by each individual for himself (pp. 90–91).

Understanding people from this perspective can be achieved through different types of phenomenological analysis (see for example Bartjes, 1991). The different analysis procedures used share a common goal of trying to study human experience from the point of view of the person being studied, in a careful and detailed fashion.

The problem of 'bracketing' in analysing what people say

In an earlier section the importance of 'bracketing' or setting aside personal assumptions in phenomenological analysis was discussed. The methodology developed by Husserl may be characterized by the phrase 'back to the things themselves'— the study of 'everyday experience as expressed in everyday language ... the realm of naive experience' (Valle *et al.*, 1989, p. 9), and a crucial process in this method is bracketing. The process of bracketing ensures that the assumptions, values, beliefs and theories that the researcher may hold, do not *distort* or *change* the meaning of what the respondent said during the interview. This is true throughout all stages of a study, but it is particularly crucial at the point of analysis.

However, the use of bracketing in studies where an existential perspective is used raises some problems for the researcher. The personal views and opinions of the researcher that may be regarded as 'prejudices' when bracketing is called for, have in fact elicited the researcher's interest in that particular 'experience' in the first place. Consequently these personal perspectives have already played a role in shaping the form and content of the data that have emerged in any qualitative study using this approach. The personal concerns of the researcher have become an important influential element on the study.

The need to be able to recognize the biases and prejudices of the researcher cannot be 'achieved by bracketing or forgetting all our pre-judgements and prejudices' (Bernstein, 1983, p. 138), because these personal concerns and orientations play an important role in the research itself. These 'biases' often help to identify more clearly what the important issues are or what questions need to be addressed. However, it is certainly possible to suspend some of our more obvious biases (or personal interests, agendas, beliefs). Being aware of bias can minimize its impact on our understanding and interpretation (Spinelli, 1989).

Kvale (1983) wrote about the 'essential tension' between a state of having no interest in a particular 'experience' whatsoever and the need to be sensitive to the topic of the interview. He conceded that the process of total bracketing was an ideal rather than a realistic possibility. Moreover, he suggested that the researcher requires both some knowledge of the area being studied and the ability to set aside personal prejudices in order to allow new facets of the experience to emerge from the interview data. Hycner (1985) recommended that researchers list explicitly all of the 'personal and/or situational factors' that may influence the research in order to overcome this very real problem. Every researcher starts an investigation with some knowledge or assumptions about the area to be studied.

The structure of the 'lifeworld'

The lifeworld is the world of experience as it is lived. Van den Berg (1972a) described the key areas that must be addressed when seeking an understanding of another person's lifeworld. He described four major domains:

- the relationship between the individual and his or her *worldly environment*
- the relationship between the individual and his or her *body*
- the individual's life history in *time* and
- the *communication* that occurs between people.

People constantly refer to these aspects of the lifeworld because they provide a way of structuring personal experiences in a meaningful way and of relating them to other people. In many ways they provide a basis for communicating with other people and understanding them. Most people think about great or difficult 'times' in their lives, remember traumatic events or anticipate pleasant experiences in the future. People note many details about the 'important' places they have been to when on holiday or through different work experiences.

In addition, we continually refer to the other people who shared or participated in our experiences. We think about the way our bodies reacted to particular events or people. These four aspects lead on to a fifth aspect of the lifeworld that was not explicitly mentioned by Van den Berg, and that is the individual's *sense of self*. These aspects form the basis for exploring the experiences of another person.

Phenomenologically based healthcare research

In drawing our attention to the merits of a phenomenological approach to research Keen (1975) wrote:

Phenomenology does not yield new information in the way that science pushes back the frontiers of knowledge. Its task is less to give us new ideas than to make explicit those ideas, assumptions, and implicit presuppositions upon which we already behave and experience life. Its task is to reveal to us exactly what we already know and that we know it, so that we can be less puzzled about ourselves. Were it to tell us something that we did not know, it would not be telling us anything about ourselves, and therefore it would not be important (p. 18).

Van Manen (1990) expressed a similar point of view as follows:

So phenomenology does not offer us the possibility of effective theory with which we can now explain and/or control the world, but rather it offers us the possibility of plausible insights that bring us in more direct contact with the world (p. 9).

The phenomenological approach is very different from the traditional approach used in much social science research. Phenomenology is an attempt to really get to know how another person is experiencing the world. Such an endeavour has the potential to be especially useful in professional helping and caring relationships.

Kestenbaum (1982a) argued a case for the use of phenomenologically based healthcare research on the grounds that it provided a powerful set of techniques for exploring patient and professional viewpoints. He suggested that these could be used to reshape professional practice and policies because the approach offered a:

... perspective for the elucidation of the experience and reality of illness and that illness as it is *lived through* by the patient...the existential meaning of illness, of illness-as-lived, and to address issues pertinent to such an understanding and perspective (Kestenbaum, 1982a, pp. vii–viii).

Another possible advantage of the phenomenological perspective in research studies may be found in the opportunities that it offers for the development of a diverse range of understandings of 'illness', 'health' and 'healthcare workers'. On another occasion Kestenbaum (1982b) argued that:

> ... phenomenology can help the culture of medicine and health care to expand the ways in which it thinks about the phenomenon of illness; it can insistently remind health professionals that illness is an experience and is intelligible as an experience. This experiential perspective makes it possible for phenomenology to elucidate illness both in its personal, individual manifestations and in its general or universal expressions ... Thus, the promise of phenomenology ... is not limited to its use in improving patient care. In grasping the intelligibility of illness as a lived experience, phenomenology helps us to understand something about ourselves, our possibilities and our limitations (p. 16).
>
> A phenomenological sense clearly is fundamental to most care-giving and helping functions typically associated with nursing, and for this reason it is not surprising that nurses traditionally have been concerned with how the sick experience their world (p. 21).

The phenomenological approach has gradually gained wider acceptance in the field of qualitative health research and in qualitative nursing research in particular. Several advocates of the approach in nursing have described in great detail some of possibilities and the pitfalls of the phenomenological perspective (see for example Omery, 1983; Watson, 1985; Drew, 1986; Swanson-Kauffmann and Schonwald, 1988; Morse, 1989; Holmes, 1990; Bartjes, 1991; Wilkes, 1991). Some of the theoretical frameworks for nursing practice have been developed from a phenomenological viewpoint; Benner and Wrubel (1989), Paterson and Zderad (1988) and Watson (1979, 1985) have all described approaches to nursing care that are grounded in existential phenomenology.

One very early example of this approach that involved nurses was a study of professional socialization by Olesen and Whittaker (1968). They used a phenomenological perspective to demonstrate how the 'uninteresting world of everyday living' (the silent dialogue) had a powerful influence over the nursing culture that helped to shape the attitudes and behaviours of students throughout the duration of their nursing training. In contrast, a very recent example of the approach in action was provided by Gullickson (1993) in her study of peoples' experiences of 'living with chronic illness'. The approach used in both of these studies was grounded in phenomenology, although the ways in which the data were collected and analysed differed.

More popular, but nevertheless informative and stimulating applications of the approach may be found in the work of Sacks (1985) and Kleinman (1988). Sacks has attempted to bridge the gap between the fields of neurology and psychology by developing a psychological understanding of the impact of neurological illness on his patients. The focus of Kleinman's work was to 'discover' the psychological impact of chronic disease on patients and their families in an effort to help them cope more effectively. Both of these writers have provided more 'popular' as opposed to research-based accounts of peoples' experiences that are moving and edifying accounts of the lives of patients and physicians.

Some limitations of the phenomenological approach

A number of important criticisms have been levelled at the approach. Perhaps the only 'generalization' that may be confidently made about the phenomenological approach is that the findings 'cannot be generalized' to a wider population. Each year millions of patients are treated in clinics and hospitals and therefore the findings from the 10 patients described here cannot reflect the experiences of so many other people.

However, the usefulness of the findings from this type of study may be gauged when nurses and patients read and consider the findings carefully. Van Manen (1990) referred to the 'phenomenological nod' response that may be used to evaluate a piece of phenomenological research as follows: '... a good phenomenological description is something that we can nod to, recognising it as an experience that we have had or could have had' (p. 27).

A second major limitation of phenomenology lies in the expected outcomes from any study underpinned by this approach. Phenomenologically based studies aim to *describe* rather than *explain why* certain types of experiences have occurred (Neyle and West, 1991). However, this may be perceived as a strength rather than a weakness. It depends on the particular perspective that a person wishes to assume.

A third limitation is the rather 'difficult language' and the complexities of the methods used to analyse data. Neyle and West (1991) suggested that these factors are likely to preclude the uptake of the phenomenological approach by practising nurses for the foreseeable future.

Some background details about the interviews with patients

As part of a larger study to explore the 'caring relationship' that exists between nurses and patients in hospital, qualitative interviews with 10 patients in a general hospital were arranged. Six men and four women took part in the study. The patients were selected from medical and surgical wards. The major criteria for selecting patients were that they had to have been in hospital for several days and be well enough to be interviewed in a side ward where minimum disruptions could be guaranteed. Patients were selected in consultation with the nurses in charge of the ward.

Patients were asked to talk about their experiences of being cared for in as much detail as possible. During the interviews, patients were encouraged to expand fully on the things they said through the use of open questions. Patients related their thoughts and feelings as well as details about the social setting in which 'care' was experienced. A small number of standard questions was used to get patients to talk about:

- what the nurses did and how they did their work
- the type of relationship that developed between the nurses and the patients
- how patients perceived caring acts or caring individuals and
- what, if anything, the patients gave to the nurses.

The patients were aged between 28 and 70 years. The ward staff helped to identify patients who would act as 'respondents' or 'informants' in the study. The nature of the study was explained fully and voluntary participation was obtained. Only one patient who agreed initially to take part did not do so; she was discharged unexpectedly. It should be emphasized that the patients who become informants for the research were people who were willing to share their experiences with me. Especially 'articulate' individuals were not sought out—although this is a tactic often used in phenomenological investigations to ensure that very detailed descriptions of a particular phenomenon are obtained. The emphasis was on 'ordinary' people who were patients at the time.

The purpose of the study and how each patient came to be selected was made clear to all potential informants. Assurances were given that whatever was said during the interviews was confidential and the informant could not be identified in any reports of the study. It was suggested that there were no 'right' or 'wrong' answers because the questions were designed to get people to express their personal views, opinions and experiences. Informants were encouraged to interrupt the interview at any time to seek clarification about any matter. All patients were asked to give their consent to the interview and to the tape recording.

The interviews lasted about 45 minutes on average. They were taped with a small hand-held recorder. All the informants seemed comfortable with the recorder, which did not appear to intrude on the interview process. After each interview, impressionistic notes about the interviews and the patients were logged on the same day. In addition, each recording was listened to and a provisional analysis was undertaken on the day of the interview. This initial analysis was recommended by Lofland and Lofland (1984). After analysing 10 interviews it was apparent that no radically new ideas were emerging from the data.

Some months later the interviews were transcribed word for word. This was a lengthy and laborious process which allowed me to become very well acquainted with each patient's account of their experiences. The initial analysis and impressionistic notes completed on the day of the interview helped to rekindle detailed images of each individual patient during the final and in-depth analysis. The tapes were also used at this stage of the analysis. Interviewing patients in the immediate ward setting helped to contextualize the experiences, making them more current and tangible, but it was sometimes difficult to ensure that interruptions did not occur. The patients were very disclosing.

A full and detailed account of the methodological stages involved in the analysis of the interviews has been provided elsewhere together with a complete transcript of one interview analysed from beginning to end (Morrison, 1991, 1992). These sources will prove useful for researchers interested in using this approach in their work.

Four major themes accounted for the patients' experiences and these have been described separately in Chapters 4–7. The themes were as follows:

- patients experienced crushing vulnerability
- patients adopted a particular mode of self-presentation
- patients evaluated the services provided in hospital
- patients' personal concerns assumed great importance.

The patients

The patients who took part in the study were inpatients in a large teaching hospital:

- Florence (55) had spent only 3 days in hospital, but she had had several earlier experiences as a patient. She had 'blind faith' in the doctors and nurses and became emotional during the interview as she described her husband's death.
- James (67) was a retired headteacher and had spent 1 full week in hospital undergoing a series of tests. He had also been an inpatient on previous occasions. He was very conscious of the need to set out the 'boundaries' for his relationships with others while in hospital.
- Eileen (61), a recently diagnosed diabetic, had spent a full week in hospital after being brought into hospital as an emergency admission after she collapsed at home. She was very keen to talk and very positive in her attitude about the hospital and the staff.
- Tim (48) had spent several weeks in the hospital and had been transferred to another hospital for specialist treatment during his admission. When he was in hospital he discovered he had lung cancer and at one point he thought that he also had secondary growths. After a series of investigations he received treatment for a kidney cyst. Tim spoke freely about his condition and mentioned that he had taken Valium and antidepressants over the years. He really wanted to talk despite the fact that he was a very nervous person.

- Hugh (28) had spent a week in hospital undergoing a series of tests that resulted in surgery. He provided a very negative account of his stay in hospital and felt that he was treated like an 'object' rather than a person. He felt as though he had no control over what was happening.

- George (62) had had several previous admissions to hospital and on this occasion he was in hospital for 7 days. He did not have a lot of direct nursing care, but was being prepared for surgery later in the week. He was rather shy and introverted, but watched how the staff dealt with other patients who were very ill and unstable medically.

- Martha (35) stayed in hospital for 8 weeks because she needed extensive skin surgery. She had come down from the north of England because the surgeon in this hospital was the 'top man' for this type of surgery. She needed two operations and had to stay in hospital much longer than was originally planned. Her mother was ill too and her husband could only visit at the weekend. She was very lonely and tearful.

- Zoe (57) needed skin surgery and was in hospital for 3 weeks. She had come down from the north of England for this specialist treatment. Unlike Martha, she seemed to cope better with being away from home.

- Ed (70) needed surgery on his pancreas because he was in great pain. He had been in hospital for 3 weeks at the time of the interview. He seemed lonely and very concerned about his companion who visited him every day. He was recovering well and was now fully mobile.

- Al (67) had returned to hospital for more surgery. On his last visit he discovered that he had cancer and he knew that it could be 'terminal'. The cancer had now returned following surgery and he needed to have another operation to remove it. He disclosed many details about himself and described how he and his family might cope with the unpredictable future.

Summary

The sketch provided above is an oversimplification and must be treated as an introduction only. The interested reader must follow-up these ideas in the much more detailed accounts provided elsewhere. If this account serves as a stimulus to encourage you to seek out more advanced descriptions of the phenomenological approach then it will have been a success.

The existential–phenomenological approach outlined above guided the approach to interviews and analysis with nurses and patients in a hospital setting. As the book unfolds, the interviews with patients are considered against a context of some broader psychological theories. Readers will come to see how both researchers and practitioners can find the phenomenological approach rewarding. Practitioners may find that one of the major advantages of this approach is that it can help carers to develop an in-depth understanding of the patients in a professional care setting.

Further reading

Anderson, J.M. (1989) The phenomenological perspective. In: J.M. Morse (ed.) *Qualitative Nursing Research. A Contemporary Dialogue*. Aspen, Rockville, Maryland, pp. 15–26.

Bartjes, A. (1991) Phenomenology in clinical practice. In: G. Gray and M. Pratt (eds) *Towards a Discipline of Nursing*. Churchill Livingstone, Melbourne, pp. 247–264.

Charmaz, K. (1990) 'Discovering' chronic illness: using grounded theory. *Social Science and Medicine*, 30 (11), 1161–1172.

Giorgi, A. (1970) *Psychology as a Human Science: A Phenomenologically Based Approach*. Harper and Row, New York.

Keen, E. (1975) *A Primer in Phenomenological Psychology*.

Holt, Rinehart and Winston, New York (reprinted in 1982 by University Press of America, Lanham).

May, R. (1960) *Existential Psychology*. Random House, New York.

Polkinghorne, D. (1989) Phenomenological research methods. In: R.S. Valle and S. Halling (eds) *Existential–Phenomenological Perspectives in Psychology. Exploring the Breadth of Human Experience*. Plenum Press, New York, pp. 41-60.

Spinelli, E. (1989) *The Interpreted World: An Introduction to Phenomenological Psychology*. Sage, London.

Stevenson, L. (1987) *Seven Theories of Human Nature*, 2nd edn. Oxford University Press, Oxford.

Wilkes, L. (1991) Phenomenology: a window to the nursing world. In: G. Gray and M. Pratt (eds) *Towards a Discipline of Nursing*. Churchill Livingstone, Melbourne, pp. 229-246.

Chapter 3

A psychological view of the patients' world

Here then is the paradox. We have a group of people who have come into an occupation because they wish to work with and help people, yet they wait until people are sick before offering this help. Not only that, but they allow organisational factors, desire for status and fear of involvement to ensure that although tasks may be done to people, whatever happens they will not get involved with them (Chapman, 1983).

Introduction

The previous chapter explored some of the basic principles of phenomenological psychology and suggested that the approach is particularly useful in helping to develop a fuller understanding of a person's view of the world as a researcher and/or practising clinician. In this chapter several of the important psychological theories that have been described in the literature are outlined since these may help us to become more aware of some of the issues that influence patients' and nurses' experiences. In many research studies, the research that has already been reported shapes the research questions that new researchers ask. A wide range of theories about 'patients' could have been chosen. Instead, the theories discussed in this chapter are highly selective and have proved useful and helpful in other research contexts and in the teaching of psychology to nursing students.

Learned helplessness

The theory of learned helplessness was described by Martin Seligman (1975, 1992; Seligman *et al.*, 1979) following experiments with animals. In a typical experiment in the laboratory, an animal (a dog or rat) was placed in a special cage with a wire mesh floor. The animal is given electric shocks and the rate, duration and strength of the shocks were determined by the researcher. All changes in the animal's behaviour were observed over time and recorded. At the start of the experiment the animals were observed to react frantically to the shocks— running around, jumping, squealing and so on. As the experiment continued over time, typical changes in the animal's behaviour were observed. The animal *learned* that it can do little to escape the dreadful conditions in the cage and eventually makes no attempt to escape from the cage. Many experimental animals became very anxious and developed ulcers.

Subtle differences in the animal's behaviour were observed as changes in the experimental conditions were made. When the animal had a reliable predictor that a shock was imminent, such as a light in the cage coming on, they responded with fear only when a danger signal was present. If on the other hand they had no *reliable predictor* of danger the animals displayed anxious behaviour continuously. It appeared that being able to *predict* unpleasant environmental circumstances made those awful circumstances somewhat more tolerable. Those experimental animals who were provided with stimuli that reliably predicted danger were found to be healthier and lived longer than animals that did not have such a stimulus. In other words 'helplessness is the psychological state that frequently results when events are uncontrollable' (Seligman, 1975, p. 9).

Seligman suggested that the learned helplessness model could be a useful model for understanding depression in humans. Of course there are real difficulties with extrapolating the findings of animal studies to human subjects. We could not set up similar experiments with humans—even if people were willing to take part in such an experiment, ethical approval would not be given because of the pain and suffering involved. However, Seligman noted similarities between his laboratory experiments and other 'natural' experiments. He described how some American soldiers in Vietnam survived torture while others became ill and died. The two groups of soldiers differed in one important respect. One group never gave up hoping and believing that they would eventually be rescued, while those who became ill and died lost this hope. They came to believe that no matter what they did they would not survive, they had no control over the environment in which they found themselves. This application of the model introduced a 'cognitive' element into the theory of learned helplessness.

Assuming that the theory can be applied to humans we know that learned helplessness can affect different aspects of a person's life. It can:

- disrupt the ability to learn
- produce emotional disorder
- produce physical symptoms such as anxiety and stomach ulcers
- result in death.

Institutionalized helplessness in hospital

One further application of the theory refers to ways people respond to hospitalization. People who come into hospital because they are ill receive treatment and care. They give up their independence to a greater or lesser degree and are subject to the authority of the doctors and nurses managing their care. Just like a child, the patient is relieved of *responsibility* while at the same time he or she loses the freedom to make decisions about their lives. This may be very frustrating for the person, particularly if they are in hospital for a lengthy period. It often leads to changes in behaviour. The frustration is displayed in many different forms. A nurse may become a target for bitter criticism or an 'angel of mercy' in the eyes of patients.

A number of social scientists have pointed out that hospitals, like other institutional settings, may have a profound and damaging effect on the people who live in them (Goffman, 1968). The influence of the institution is particularly telling when a person has been in hospital for long-term care, such as the severely mentally ill or other individuals with chronic disease or disabilities. The staff have the *power* and *authority* to influence greatly the existence of the residents. The patients' lives are regulated by routines, rules and practices often designed to meet the needs of the staff. Patients can become *helpless* in this situation. They learn that no matter how hard they try to take control over their lives, the staff continue to dictate any changes in their existence under the guise of the professional helping role. Thus:

> Institutional systems are all too often insensitive to their inhabitants' need for control over important events. The usual doctor–patient relationship is not designed to provide the patient with a sense of control. The doctor knows all, and usually tells little; the patient is expected to sit back 'patiently' and rely on professional help. While such extreme dependency may be helpful to certain patients in some circumstances, a greater degree of control would help others … This loss of control may further weaken a physically sick person and cause death. (Seligman, 1975 pp. 182–183).

The learned helplessness scenario sounds rather sinister and unreal but Seligman has drawn on a wide range of anecdotal evidence and several studies of institutionalized residents to support this position (Lefcourt, 1973; Schulz and Aderman, 1974). Nurses and other healthcare workers 'care' for people and do not set out deliberately to harm them or hinder their recovery. The workings of institutions are complex and the process of learned helplessness can be fostered by staff unknowingly and unwillingly. As we will see in later chapters, people (as patients) respond differently to the ways in which staff care for them. Some of these responses are healthy and adaptive; others are not.

Caring for people in an institutional context can alter the way both the staff and the patients behave. Menzies (1970) provided an early example of how the work situation can influence the relationships between nurses and patients. She described a scenario in which the hospital culture ensured that contact between nurses and patients is minimized. The net result is that nurses steer clear of the strong emotional reactions that patients sometimes express as a natural response to their circumstances. The position of nurses in the work setting means that they can be exposed to the risks of emotional outbursts—fearfulness, anger, loss, grief and embarrassment—all of which are difficult to deal with even for experienced nurses. Menzies suggested that the hospital culture that encourages nurses to avoid these sorts of 'emotional' patients acts as a 'defence against anxiety' in staff throughout the hospitalized system of care.

Menzies described a number of working patterns that support her opinions. The relationship between the nurse and the patient is broken up and there is a greater emphasis on the 'tasks' that have to be done rather than on the person who is ill. People as patients become depersonalized. They become the 'appendicitis in the side ward'. There is a complete denial of the emotional aspects of human behaviour in both staff and patients. The performance of the nursing tasks becomes 'ritualistic'. It is true that a number of developments in care have helped to lessen the negative effects of this sort of hospital culture, but the effectiveness of recent developments should not be overestimated. A brief talk with patients, friends or relatives who have attended hospital recently will remind you of how much development work still needs to be done. There is still a long way to go to achieve the high standard of care that patients deserve. The emotional side of the nurses' role remains an important facet of nursing today (Smith, 1992).

In addition, Cassee (1975) claimed that there was a need for much more research if nurses were to develop an accurate understanding of the relationships between professional carers and patients. We still know very little about the complexities of nurse–patient relationships almost 20 years on and there is still a need for in-depth studies of this relationship. Cassee suggested, however, that the research at that time indicated:

> ... that behaviour that is conducive to the healing process— 'therapeutic behaviour'—has some special characteristics. Apparently, the patient's most positive reactions are obtained in a situation aiming at an *open two-way communication between therapist* (either physician or nurse) *and patient.* This open communication consists of at least two elements. In the first place, it includes informing the patient about the nature and seriousness of his illness, the treatment procedures to be followed, and the general rules prevailing in the hospital. The fact that this information must be compatible with the needs of the patient proved to be the main problem...It is necessary to know what is worrying the patient. Consequently, the second element in communication with the patient is to encourage him to express his anxieties, thus enabling him to take part in the decision-making concerning his treatment (Cassee, 1975, p. 225).

Healthcare professionals expect patients to assume greater responsibility for their own health and care yet we as professional carers fail to foster an attitude of independence when these people come into professional arenas. Following a small study of patient collaboration using the grounded theory approach, Waterworth and Luker (1990) identified a major theme in the patients' perspective as 'toeing the line'. That is, they are more concerned with being perceived by the professionals as 'good' patients than participating in decision-making about their care and treatment. If people respond to the ways they define social situations (discussed more fully below), then the cues that they use to arrive at such a definition must be provided by the other people in that context. If patients are 'reluctant collaborators' (Waterworth and Luker, 1990), then the staff in the hospital may be working in ways that favour this social perception of the patient world.

The process of learned helplessness reveals several implications for the work of the nurse. First, the nurse has a very important role in promoting independence in ill people. This can only be done successfully if the nurse is knowledgeable about the ways institutions work and how people (both the professionals and their patients) respond to particular circumstances and working environments. Second, the nurse also needs to evaluate *why* things are done in a certain way. She needs to ask if rules, routines and decisions are for the benefit of the staff or the patient. This can be an especially challenging activity for professional carers. We often assume that we know what is best for our patients. In many cases this is so, but sometimes it is not.

Third, the nurse needs to be aware of the often devastatingly harmful effects of institutions on individuals and particularly the patient group. Patients may become more dependent, likely to stay in hospital longer and fail to comply with health education advice and treatment. This is especially important with some groups of patients such as the elderly, the long-term ill (both adults and children), the mentally ill and the mentally handicapped (see for example Miller, 1985).

Finally, this area highlights the importance of the nurse's role in providing information to patients. A large number of research studies have clearly demonstrated the positive results of providing clear information to patients in a simple and supportive manner. Devine and Cook (1983) provided evidence in the form of a meta-analysis of 49 research studies designed to study the effects of giving information to surgical patients pre-operatively. In addition, the provision of information to parents has also been shown to positively affect children in care (Skipper and Leonard, 1968; Ferguson, 1979). However, this information must be given in such a way that it actively encourages the patient to have more control and predictability over his or her life. Withholding information from patients may benefit the staff and may ensure that patients do not ask more searching questions:

> Giving information to patients about their illness may be seen as something which patients do not need to know, would probably not understand anyway, might cause an emotional reaction which would interfere with their instrumental care and cure, and at the very least takes the time of the nurses and physicians away from more important tasks (Skipper *et al.*, 1964, pp. 35–36).

The role of attributions

People constantly observe and interpret the behaviour of others. Human behaviour is a function of the person and the specific context or situation in which he or she finds themselves. We behave differently at a party with our peers compared with the way we behave when we approach the bank manager to request a loan. We dress differently, speak differently and adopt a different attitude. We change the way we behave in these different situations because we define these situations as being quite different. We usually behave in a way that coincides with our definition of any situation. At the party we think we should be enjoying ourselves so we have a few drinks, become more gregarious and adopt a cheerful attitude. At the bank we want to be seen to be responsible and serious individuals capable of fulfilling our responsibilities. Each new situation places a new set of expectations on us and we try to meet these requirements.

It is interesting to note that two people may define the situation differently even though the cues we receive are identical. The important point to note is that people react not to objective features of a situation but to the sense they make of it—their own subjective interpretation of the world and the people in it (see for example the personal construct approach of the psychologist George Kelly, 1955, 1963). This principle is closely linked with the phenomenological approach to psychology which was discussed briefly in the previous chapter.

One approach that social psychologists use to develop an understanding of the ways in which people 'construe' their view of the world is known as 'attribution theory'. Attribution theory is concerned with understanding how we attribute *causes* to our own and to other people's behaviour (Pennington, 1986). We are constantly collecting data about the world and the people we meet. We use these data to make causal attributions about ourselves and other people. If we want to know more about the ways in which people *perceive* each other we *ask* them about their views about other people in a social setting. We need to be able to understand ourselves and other people if we are to communicate effectively with them. A great deal of communication with others is based on our taken-for-granted assumptions about other people and the situation they are in. These assumptions are often the result of the attributions we make about other people.

Pennington (1986) identified three important facets of the attribution theory approach as follows:

- We constantly try to *explain* our own behaviour and that of other people. This process helps to *reduce uncertainty* about how a person will behave in the future.
- We are constantly *searching for and using information* as we attribute causes.
- We are like *naive scientists* because we are continually engaged in the business of trying to describe, explain and predict social behaviour.

The theoretical foundations of attribution theory can be found in the work of Fritz Heider (1958) and the approach is phenomenologically grounded. Heider emphasized the importance of *conscious experience* within his approach as follows:

> Our concern will be with 'surface' matters, the events that occur in everyday life on a conscious level, rather than with the unconscious processes studied by psychoanalysis in 'depth' psychology (Heider, 1958, p. 1).

Heider (1958) claimed that this common sense or naive psychology had great relevance for the scientific study of interpersonal relationships because it attempted to explore people's perceptions about the world in their own terms and legitimized these personal accounts as data deserving of scientific scrutiny. He argued that the way we attribute causes is influenced by three things:

- the characteristics of the person perceiving
- the features of the object, behaviour or person being perceived
- the social setting in which the behaviour occurs.

Think for a moment about the points made at the beginning of this section. As a naive scientist or observer in a bank or at a party you may see other people behaving in particular ways and attribute 'causes' to their actions. The same process works in other social settings including hospitals.

People attribute causes of behaviour to *persons* (internal causes) or to *situations* (external causes). Internal attributions refer to the traits or characteristics we attribute to others based on their behaviour. External attributions focus on the circumstances that cause a person to behave in a particular manner. Here is an example of how the process works. You are waiting on the station platform for your train. A train stops and a few metres down from you the door opens and a well-dressed woman falls out of the carriage onto the concrete platform. As you comprehend what has happened you find that you make attributions about what has happened. Remember the three factors mentioned above that shape your perceptions. In the first instance you may decide that the woman tripped on some ill-fitting carpet near the door, or accidentally tripped on luggage left near to the door, or the crowd of overeager football supporters pushed a little too eagerly and so on. You have attributed an external cause for the behaviour that you witnessed. It was not the woman's fault.

You may run along the platform and offer assistance with the woman's bags and help her to sit down. As you do, she thanks you profusely for your kindness. Then you notice that her speech is slurred and she smells of alcohol. She is blind drunk! Your perceptions about what has happened now changes radically and the attributions you make alter too. Now the cause of her accident is more obvious. It is her own fault because she drank too much alcohol on the train. She is to blame for this mishap. You have attributed an internal cause for the accident. You are not likely to offer much more help to this woman. You carry on waiting for your own train and leave her alone on the platform. As you gathered more information about the situation you altered your perception of what happened.

People tend to make these sorts of attributions, but they are not always so logical and straightforward. We make errors of attribution like that just mentioned. In addition some people have a tendency to attribute 'internal' causes of behaviour, while others display a tendency to attribute 'external' causes perhaps because of essential differences in personality. Some people have a strong 'locus of control' (they make internal attributions about the causes of their own behaviour) and this is especially relevant in the context of health care. Wallston and Wallston (1978) argued that people who feel themselves to be in control of their health are better able to cope with chronic illnesses compared with people who believe that the 'control' is with the professional helpers such as doctors and nurses. This perspective has been challenged by other researchers on methodological grounds. The use of questionnaires to gather data, for example, may limit the ways in which people can respond. The respondents may be given a limited number of response options and a particular structure for making attributions may be imposed (see Rogers, 1991, for a detailed critical discussion of the research). In a recent nursing text on coping with chronic illness, however, 'control' emerged as an important facet of good coping (Miller, 1992).

Attribution theory has also been used in studies of helping behaviour. Weiner (1980), for example, emphasized the mediating role that *affect* has on helping. When an individual perceives another person in need of help, he or she *attributes* the cause of this distress to internal or external factors. If *external or uncontrollable causes* of the distress have been attributed then the observer may feel sympathy and concern and is more likely to help. Think back for a moment about how you may have responded to the woman who fell out onto the train station platform. On the other hand, where an *internal or controllable cause* has been attributed the observer may feel anger or disgust and refuse to give help. There are several studies of the types of covert attributions and labels that nurses and doctors apply to particular patient groups (Jeffrey, 1979; Kelly and May, 1982). The crucial point is that people (including nurses and doctors) act in accordance with the attributions they make about patients and their relatives, and in a professional context these attributions can influence clinical judgements and decision-making in professional carers.

It has been suggested that an understanding of attribution theory can help to inform the theory of learned helplessness in humans (Abramson *et al.*, 1978). Allowing for the fact that different attribution styles exist in different people, the impact of learned helplessness on humans may be more understandable, and hence more treatable, in terms of the attributions people make about their own lives and social environments. This may be particularly relevant in long term care environments. Some psychological therapies aim explicitly at changing the type of attributions that clients make about themselves and their lives (Abramson and Martin, 1981). The goals of therapy are to re-establish a greater sense of personal control and raise self-esteem.

In reality it may be impossible for a patient to have total 'control' over a chronic illness, but patients could have some say in the type of treatment and management that is available for their remaining life. According to Seligman (1975, 1992), the institutional setting may be responsible for negative changes in the patients' behaviour and state of mind. Hence, the larger context in which attributions are made needs to be accounted for.

Doctors and nurses are also part of the institutional environment so they too have an important role to play and contribute to the process of learned helplessness. Paradoxically, doctors and nurses must promote independence in their patients if recovery and health are to be achieved. The likely outcomes of this system of care for short-stay patients and those who require long-stay care are probably quite different. Institutional care can be misguided and paternalistic (Gadow, 1980). It can unintentionally harm people through the promotion of learned helplessness.

Good and bad patients

Few people spend more than a small number of days in hospital in their lifetime yet that time can have a profound effect on the person. The fact that hospitals are total institutions (Goffman, 1968) surely has a depersonalizing effect on the individual. Perhaps the most important factor is the loss of 'control' over everyday life events (Taylor, 1979) and the

implications this loss has for the individual. In addition
'helplessness' or 'hopelessness' may provide a powerful stimulus for the carers to respond in a particular way. There is a
very real danger that nurses and doctors may actively foster
this type of learned helplessness, a point openly acknowledged
by several nurses who were interviewed in another part of this
study (Morrison, 1991, 1992).

Patients are often encouraged to be excessively compliant
and unquestioning in their approach to the staff. Several other
modes of patient self-presentation are described later. Those
who do ask questions, are in any way deviant or try to maintain
some measure of control over what is happening to them run
the risk of becoming unpopular and being 'sanctioned' by the
staff (Stockwell, 1972; Lorber, 1975). Good patients are
perceived by the staff as patients who do what they are told and
do not make trouble for the staff. This role is desirable for the
smooth running of the hospital. Cooper (1976) describes the
role as follows:

> To be a 'patient' is a unique status because one thinks it
> means that one has relinquished the right to ask questions,
> although one must accept the obligation of answering
> questions and permitting one's self to be examined. Asking
> questions seems to be the right of everyone else—especially
> physicians, strangers, and others who can deny emotional ties
> to the patient. Thoroughly exposed, the patient is expected
> patiently to submit to all manner of indignities (p. 43).

Taylor (1979) suggested that patients who submit to the good
patient role may be displaying a state of 'depressed or anxious
helplessness'.

Bad patients are seen by staff as continuously seeking
attention and information. They may be critical of the care they
receive and openly express their views. They may have to be
referred to the consultant in charge to be managed. They are
labelled as 'difficult' and are often dealt with by the most

inexperienced and junior member of the team. Their complaints may be ignored potentially with disastrous effects if the
complaints refer to important symptoms. On occasions bad
patients are tranquillized to make them more manageable
(Lorber, 1975). Stockwell (1972) collected attitudinal and
behavioural data from nurses using a variety of methods and
found that the concept of 'patient popularity' was a meaningful
term in nursing practice and influenced how the nurses interacted with patients. Unpopular patients, such as those with a
psychiatric history or patients who were themselves doctors or
nurses, were avoided or ignored. It is interesting to note that
neither 'good' nor 'bad' patients can achieve a sense of control
as patients in hospital.

There is also some evidence to suggest that physical attractiveness contributes to the perceptions of patients held by staff.
Nordholm (1980) asked 289 healthcare staff to react to stimulus photographs (attractive and unattractive individuals) by
rating the photographs on a series of bipolar rating scales. The
attractive stimulus photographs were rated more favourably
than the unattractive stimulus photographs on 12 of the 15
characteristics supplied by the researcher. Nordholm took these
results as evidence of the 'beautiful is good' stereotype that
exists amongst professional healthcare workers. Finally, our
perceptions of patients can lead to patients displaying the very
types of behaviour we expect—our perceptions become self-
fulfilling prophecies (Abraham and Shanley, 1992).

The sick role and illness behaviour

The third major area examined in this chapter was developed in
sociology, but it is nevertheless related to the earlier sections
and helps us to understand how patients and staff play different
roles in the professional setting. Talcott Parsons, a sociologist,
outlined how the 'sick role' has four major aspects (Parsons,

1951). The first is the *exemption from normal social role responsibilities*. This means that the sick person is freed up from work or other areas of life throughout the duration of the illness. The degree to which a person becomes exempt depends on the nature and severity of the illness. Moreover, a further requirement is that the illness is validated or legitimized by others (such as doctors) to prevent people from abusing the rights of the sick person.

The second aspect of the sick role is the *recognition that the person is not to blame for the illness*. The person cannot simply pull themselves together or change their attitude with a return to normal health. They cannot help the fact that they are ill. Each sick person needs to be helped and cared for if they are to get over the illness. The third aspect of the sick role deals with the motivation of the sick person. It should be clear that the unwell person *perceives the sick role as undesirable* and *is obliged to want to get well* and leave the sick role. The attribution process is at work here. Staff, and medical staff in particular, are in a position where they have to make judgements about people. They can legitimize the patient's condition. They can decide on the patient's motivational state. The nature of the care given to patients is often guided by these judgements (see Jeffrey, 1979; May and Kelly, 1982, for examples of how this process works in practice).

The fourth aspect is the *obligation to seek technically competent help* for the condition. Once this is done, the patient fulfilling the sick role must cooperate fully with the professional treatment plan so that the professional role and the sick role become complementary. These four aspects of the sick role are essentially two rights and two responsibilities— the rights include the exemption from normal responsibilities and the recognition that the ill person is not to blame for the illness, and the obligations include a desire to get well and to seek out qualified medical help.

The patient must 'perform' this role. If the patient does

not then he or she may be labelled as a 'bad patient' as follows:

> The patients who fail to conform to the sick role are considered to be 'bad patients'. When a patient fails to conform, the legitimacy of the illness itself is often questioned—that is, the patient may be suspected of malingering. An uncooperative patient may be denied continuation of hospitalisation by premature discharge because the physicians become angry with him for not living up to the fourth expectation. A convalescing patient who repeatedly complains of minor symptoms is seen as not fulfilling the third expectation to regard the sick role as an undesirable one that should be relinquished as soon as possible. This may even tempt the physician to withdraw legitimization of the sick role from such a patient. Some patients, on the other hand, may foster approved prolongation of the sick role by being 'good' patients, that is by extreme cooperativeness (sometimes even volunteering to participate in experimental procedures) (Leigh and Reiser, 1980, p. 17).

The acceptance of the sick role is influenced by several factors and not every patient assumes the role. Some illnesses are generally perceived as less acceptable by society—some sexually transmitted diseases and mental illnesses are stigmatized. A good example here is the person who attempts suicide and ends up in an accident and emergency department for initial treatment (Jeffrey, 1979).

The theory of the sick role does not cover all types of illness and patients. Minor conditions, incurable illness from which there is no recovery, and physical and mental handicap are three major areas of exclusion (Leigh and Reiser, 1980). In addition there is the growing tendency in medicine to *attribute responsibility* for certain types of illness to patients themselves. Smoking, being overweight and a lack of exercise are seen as important factors that contribute to illness. They are also areas of the patient's life for which he or she is solely responsible. Some medical and surgical teams now refuse to treat people unless they play their role by altering certain life patterns—stopping smoking, losing weight and taking regular exercise. Unfortunately, it is much easier to tell people what they should do than it is to get them to do it.

It may also be more accurate to say that individuals are only *partly responsible* for these personal 'deficiencies'—a great deal of advertising is aimed at getting people to eat, drink and smoke more, and to be entertained passively by watching television and home videos. In addition, peer pressure can be very influential and can help people to change their lifestyles. However, it can also have a negative effect. It may be extremely difficult to go home after a consultation with a surgeon and stop smoking before an operation, when all the other people in the home smoke too and have no intention of stopping. These factors place a very heavy burden on the person who has to change their lifestyle before receiving care and treatment.

Summary

The three areas examined in this chapter can help us to understand why patients, and the professionals looking after them behave as they do. The theories outlined here are, however, only partially correct. There is a need to examine the world of the patient more carefully to gain a clearer understanding of the social setting in which care and treatment are administered. The theories described above can then be evaluated as ways of representing the patients' world and as teaching aids for healthcare workers . In the following chapters the experiences of a small sample of patients are described in depth by using the phenomenological approach to psychology described in Chapter 2.

Further reading

Aronson, E. (1988) *The Social Animal*, 5th edn. Freeman, New York.

Baron, R.A. and Byrne, D. (1987) *Social Psychology: Understanding Human Interaction*, 5th edn. Allyn and Bacon, Boston.

Burns, R.B. (1991) *Essential Psychology: For Students and Professionals in the Health and Social Services*, 2nd edn. Kluwer, London.

Goffman, E. (1968) *Asylums: Essays on the Social Situation of Mental Patients and Other Inmates*. Harmondsworth, Penguin.

Jeffrey, R. (1979) Normal rubbish: deviant patients in casualty departments. *Sociology of Health and Illness*, 1 (1), 90–107.

Kelly, M.P. and May, P. (1982) Good and bad patients: a review of the literature and a theoretical critique. *Journal of Advanced Nursing*, 7, 147–156.

May, D. and Kelly, M.P. (1982) Chancers, pests and poor wee souls: problems of legitimation in psychiatric nursing. *Sociology of Health and Illness*, 4 (3), 279–301.

Miller, J.F. (1992) *Coping with Chronic Illness. Overcoming Powerlessness*, 2nd edn. F.A. Davis, Philadelphia.

Rogers, W.S. (1991) *Explaining Health and Illness. An Exploration of Diversity*. Harvester Wheatsheaf, London.

Rosenhan, D.L. (1973) On being sane in insane places. *Science*, 179, 250–258.

Schank, M.J. and Lawrence, D.M. (1993) Young adult women: lifestyle and health locus of control. *Journal of Advanced Nursing*, 18, 1235–1241.

Seligman, M.E.P. (1975) *Helplessness: On Depression, Development, and Death*. Freeman, New York (re-issued in 1992).

Skevington, S. (ed.) (1984) *Understanding Nurses: The Social Psychology of Nursing*. Wiley, Chichester.

Swain, J. (1989) Learned helplessness theory with people with learning difficulties: the psychological price of powerlessness. In: A. Brechin and J. Walmsley (eds) *Making Connections. Reflecting on the Lives and Experiences of People with Learning Difficulties*. Hodder and Stoughton, London.

Zinder-Wernet, P. and Weiss, S. (1987) Health locus of control and preventive health behaviour. *Western Journal of Nursing Research*, 9, 160–179.

Chapter 4

Patients experienced 'crushing vulnerability'

The experience of hospital in-patient care not only gives rise to feelings of fear and anxiety but often also produces a sense of depersonalization, or loss of self-identity ... this type of depersonalisation stems from the loss of the patient's normal social roles and separation from their familiar environment. It is accentuated by the impersonality of hospital care, with patients often feeling that they have been treated as 'just another case' rather than as individuals with their own feelings, concerns and experiences (Morgan, 1991).

Introduction

Some background details about the study and the patients who took part in the study were provided in Chapter 2. In Chapters 4–7 the findings from the interviews with patients are described and discussed. In this chapter one of the major themes to characterize the patients' experience of 'being cared for' in a hospital setting is described. Patients experienced 'crushing vulnerability' during their time in hospital. The emotional upheaval and uncertainty that are part of being ill and in a strange and frightening place raised all sort of issues and questions for the patients who took part in the study. The vulnerable position of the patient means that he or she may become very dependent. As nurses we must ask what we can do to help patients get through this difficult time in hospital.

Organization and layout of the theme

The theme 'patients experienced crushing vulnerability' has
been organized in a particular way to ensure that it is described
fully and clearly. Under the major heading 'Patients experienced crushing vulnerability', several subthemes are described.
These subthemes collectively convey different aspects of the
experience of crushing vulnerability. Examples of subthemes
described in this chapter are: (a) The hospital environment was
strange; (b) Anxiety about being treated like an object; (c)
Positive impact of being treated like a person; (d) Shattering
impact of cancer; (e) Traumatic investigations and surgery; (f)
Cancelled operation was a major setback; and (g) Anxious
suspicion.

Very fine discriminations between patients, or for the same
patient on different occasions, are contained in some of these
subthemes and therefore a third level of organization has been
used occasionally. For example, in subtheme (b) the following
subheadings have been used to illustrate different aspects of
this subtheme: 'Ignored during the handovers', and 'Public
discussion of personal details was embarrassing'. An example
of the organizing structure is represented in Figure 1.

The findings presented in Chapters 5–7 are also laid out in
the same way. In addition, verbatim extracts from the interviews have occasionally been included as evidence to support a
particular point and to give a flavour of the interviews as a
whole—what people said and how they described their experiences. These extracts have been enclosed within double quota-
tion marks to emphasize that they represent the very personal
accounts of the patients who took part in the study.

PATIENTS EXPERIENCED CRUSHING VULNERABILITY

Patients experienced being cared for during a time of crushing
vulnerability. The emotional upheaval of being ill and in

PATIENTS EXPERIENCED CRUSHING VULNERABILITY (Level 1, major theme, bold capitals)

(a) The hospital environment was strange (Level 2, subtheme, alphabetically ordered)
(b) Anxiety about being treated like an object

Ignored during handovers (Level 3, very fine discrimination, italic lettering)
Public discussion of personal details was embarrassing

(c) Positive impact of being treated like a person
(d) Shattering impact of cancer
(e) Traumatic investigations and surgery
(f) Cancelled operation was a major setback
(g) Anxious suspicion

Figure 1 Organization of the qualitative themes.

hospital set the scene. The things that nurses and doctors did for the patients and the way in which these things were done conveyed to the patient a feeling of being cared for. Sometimes patients felt both cared for and uncared for during their stay in hospital through the actions and sensitivities of the staff.

(a) The hospital environment was strange
The hospital environment was experienced as a daunting place for a number of patients. It was unpleasant, big, strange and nerve racking. This strange environment led some patients to become acutely aware of their own vulnerability and uncertainty about what they should do in this strange place. James, an elderly man and formerly a head school teacher, stated:

> "I don't like being in a situation that I don't know what to do".

Zoe was frightened and wondered what would happen to her. She could not anticipate the future, and had no control over her situation now. She had to rely on the staff. In hospital, strange people came to talk to her and to take blood samples. It seemed correct to let strangers do intimate things. Other patients did not like being in hospital and were there because they had to be there—James did not like hospital and he felt that he was there under duress.

Some patients were better able to cope with the hospital environment. They adapted to the strange environment and came to see it as less intimidating than others did. This is particularly so for those patients who had several admissions to hospital or who stayed for any length of time. They became accustomed to the place. However, this is not always true. One patient, Martha, spent several weeks in hospital after extensive plastic surgery. Although she knew the staff well and felt well cared for, she found herself crying from time to time because hospital just "got to" her.

Being in hospital is a frightening experience. Patients are full of uncertainty and are unclear about what will happen to them. The unfamiliar surroundings heighten their inability to make predictions about even mundane aspects of their lives as patients. Their existence is often structured around the work of the ward. It is especially difficult to adapt to this environment at times of illness.

(b) Anxiety about being treated like an object
One of the most important, if somewhat intangible, pre-requisites in caring for people is the need to treat patients as people. Here we see how the approach that staff employ in hospital can lead to anxiety. Some patients found that being in hospital induced anxiety about being *treated like an object*. Florence had a dreadful fear of being made to feel like a number, and she recognized in herself a tendency to talk too much when she was nervous. Similarly, James also expressed his own unease and:

"...did not want to become just a name on a sheet of paper".

This is perhaps a feeling that can all too easily be generated by the staff in any hospital as they interact with patients as part of their daily work. Think for a moment about the ways we constantly refer to people in hospital as 'patients', 'schizophrenics', 'diabetics' and so on. This type of labelling is necessary to some extent, to promote a common understanding amongst staff, but it can all too easily degenerate into a type of non-person treatment that often typifies professional care. We must remind ourselves constantly that *patients are people* too.

Patients have to find ways of dealing with this anxiety. James was able to overcome this objectification process by talking to other patients. However, not all the other patients were so fortunate and there was generally a high level of disappointment with the personal side of the care the patients received during their time in hospital. Hugh was a young man in his early thirties and found that his feelings were ignored completely by staff. In particular he was:

Ignored during the handovers
The handovers between the different nursing shifts were usually conducted at the foot of Hugh's bed and he was ignored by the staff. Hugh really wanted the nurses to talk *to* him, but instead the staff talked *about* him as if he did not exist:

> "... its almost as if you're being talked about and are not there. You know 'this is Mr D. who had a bath' ... I'M HERE ...".

While being ignored was bad enough, it was made worse by the fact that:

Public discussion of personal details was embarrassing
During the handover, which was carried out in front of the patients, the distinct lack of privacy embarrassed Hugh:

> "... I don't think it should be done in front of the patient, being talked about is ... embarrassing and wasted time ...".

(c) Positive impact of being treated like a person
Not every patient experienced the high level of anxiety just mentioned. In contrast, several patients commented on the positive impact of being treated like a person. It made some patients feel better and promoted self-esteem and feelings of self-worth.

Being treated like a person promoted recovery
Some patients suggested that the feeling of being treated like a person had a positive effect on their well-being. It is widely acknowledged that psychological well-being can influence recovery rates (see for example Devine and Cook, 1983; Ley,

1988; Nichols, 1993). Although the staff did nothing spectacular for Florence they just made her:

> "... feel like a person, you know, not a number ...".

Being treated like a person helped Florence to relax and get better.

It felt good to be called by your first name

Some patients cherished the way the staff called them by their first name, but not every patient did. For some it appears that this can help the patient feel like a person, but for others it may promote feelings of unease and be interpreted as a lack of respect. In general, however, it seemed to symbolize a need to be treated like a person rather than an object or number and this view was shared by several patients. It felt good when staff knew the patient's first name and used it, though not every patient appreciated being called by their first name; for example:

> "I'd rather be called by my Christian name and I feel more at home. And I think this status of being Mrs David or Mrs Jones is past you know ... Here they call us 'Eileen' and so on ...".

One patient, Eileen, expressed the need for caution and felt that nurses should not call *all* patients by their first names; some patients, especially the older ones, don't like overfamiliarity.

Staff did not make patients feel small

The positive attitude of the staff also had an impact on patients. Staff did not make Florence feel 'small', they were friendly and treated her like a workmate, which she liked very much. Eileen felt that nurses would always respect her wishes even though they got to know her quite well and treated her like a workmate—they wouldn't overstep the mark and take advantage of her. Tim had a very positive experience when he

returned to the ward after being to another hospital for a series
of diagnostic investigations. When he came back to the ward
the nurses were genuinely glad to see him again. One of the
nurses hugged him and he really felt good:

> "When they seen me come back here last week young Jane
> got hold of me as if she hadn't seen me for donkeys years, as
> if I was a long lost brother or something. They made me feel
> like somebody ...".

(d) Shattering impact of cancer

Two of the informants who took part in the study had recently
been diagnosed as having cancer. It had a tremendous impact
on the lives of both patients. The phrase 'shattering impact of
cancer' captures the devastating effect such a diagnosis can
have on an individual and his or her family. It could also apply
equally well to other seriously disabling illness: mental illness,
disfiguring trauma or death of loved one, for example, can all
have a 'shattering impact' on a person's life.

Needed to know the truth

Both of the patients who developed cancer were in hospital for
treatment. One of their major concerns was the need to know
the truth about the condition and the possibilities or lack of
possibilities for the future. What would happen to them? How
long would they live? Would the surgery or treatment be
successful? What would happen to their families if they died?
Who would look after their families after their deaths?

Tim spoke of his need to know the worst, but none of the
doctors would tell him directly. This made him feel even more
anxious about his condition and prognosis. Eventually he was
told about his condition. He felt better after finding out the
truth, but he was very hurt because his wife was told about the
cancer before him. This meant that she was part of a 'conspiracy' and must have known he had cancer when she came to
visit him. Tim was kept in the dark. He was worried about the

burden that had been placed on her shoulders—she had to keep this secret (his cancer) to herself and could not tell him. Tim felt that she would not cope well with this. Another patient, Al, asked the professor looking after him to tell him everything.

Discovery

When Tim was eventually told he had lung cancer he went cold. He just:

"... went to pieces ...".

Gradually he came to accept the fact that he had cancer. Al was another patient who developed cancer. In the beginning it all seemed like nothing. At first he discovered a mole on his back, which was diagnosed as skin cancer after an operation. The professor told him he had cancer and it was very serious.

Thoughts about death and dying

Tim had become the subject of many teaching sessions for medical students. He saw many different doctors because of his rare condition and he thought that he was dying because so many doctors came to see him. His nervous disposition led him to think the worst because of the visits he had from medical students and different consultants. Al, on the other hand, was fearful about going into hospital in case it was terminal. When it was discovered he had cancer, it was very well developed in his body. He found himself in hospital thinking about his life:

"... life is sweet. I've got a little car, a wife and two nice children and we go and do things. Not a lot of money but it's nice. You know ... after working all your life and retiring now comes the sallow days".

He too felt that he could accept whatever was in front of him because he was older and more experienced and more accepting of things in his life.

Hope without guarantees

Although some of the patients who were interviewed had
developed a life-threatening illness, they wanted to have
'hope'. During his first operation, Al had a melanoma removed
and the operation went well, but he knew in his heart that there
were no guarantees, even though everything that could be done
surgically had been done. Some time after the first operation
another lump was discovered at outpatients and a second
operation was needed. The second operation also went well.
Now he would have to wait and see.

(e) Traumatic investigations and surgery

Lengthy and drawn-out investigations were very traumatic for
Tim, but he felt that the medical and nursing staff were
supportive. He developed high blood pressure and this was
another complication that required a move to another hospital
for specialist management. He felt much better in himself when
the blood pressure settled down. Al had to undergo two major
operations for cancer.

(f) Cancelled operation was a major setback

Tim's operation was cancelled at the last moment. All the
preparations and investigations for the operation were carried
out, but the operation was still cancelled. This was a real blow
and a further source of anxiety because Tim assumed that the
cancer had now spread to his kidneys making the operation
more dangerous. Tim calmed down after hearing that the
operation was not cancelled altogether. It was only a postpone-
ment because the doctors wanted all the results to be right
before the operation. Eventually Tim got news that the operation would proceed and he rejoiced at this news.

(g) Anxious suspicion

Tim, who discovered that he had cancer during his stay in
hospital, did not expect to be pampered and felt that if he was

pampered or the nurses spent too much time with him, he would have suspected that something was seriously amiss:

> "If they kept on I'm sure I'd think there was more wrong than is actually the case. That's how I would feel if they pampered me too much. I'd know. That I do believe".

This is a nice example of how individual patients make sense of their own particular set of circumstances. If you as a nurse want to get to know a patient well enough to make a sound and thorough clinical assessment of that patient, then you must spend time getting to know the person. In Tim's case, spending time (or as he perceived it, too much time) would only heighten his anxiety.

(h) Surrendering independence was distressing
Martha spent a long time in hospital for a series of skin graft operations. She was a young woman in her thirties and found it hard to rely on other people and give up her independence. She felt awkward at having to be helped to the toilet. She was not able to sit up after the operation and became even more dependent after the second operation. It was very distressing and upsetting:

> "... I found it very difficult, very upsetting. I really thought that after six weeks I was going back to stage one".

Gradually regained independence
Martha's independence was regained gradually, however. In the beginning the nurses had to do everything for her, such as washing, toileting and changing positions, but the nurses were able to judge what she could do for herself. Over time the staff left things ready for her and let her get on with it by herself and at her own pace. Al, on the other hand, regained his independence soon after his operations and went home quickly.

(i) Coping with bodily disfigurement was traumatic
Martha had two operations and both involved large skin grafts.
She found it very difficult to look at the operation site:

> "... and just to see it to start with was the worst bit, you feel
> like fainting ...".

However, she could not escape from the operation site and had
to accept that she had a stoma. Eventually she reached a stage
where she looked after herself again and became independent
of the staff.

(j) Difficult being away from home for a long time
Because Martha was away from her home and relatives for
such a long time, she felt as if she needed something to
compensate for being away from home. Her family could only
visit her at weekends. She was told that her surgery would take
2 or 3 weeks by her own doctor, but she had already spent 8
weeks away from her family. Martha wanted staff to spend
more time with her. Other patients on the ward made a point of
coming into her room and talking to her, and this made her feel
well supported. She also wanted the staff to talk normally to
her. The other people made her feel different in herself; they
interacted 'normally' with her. The staff were overly professional.

(k) Felt like a smelly mess compared with the nurses
Zoe messed the floor because she had diarrhoea and felt
'awful' because the student nurse had to clean it up. She
compared herself with the nurses, who were well groomed, and
felt like a smelly mess by comparison.

(l) Felt forgotten about
On one occasion Ed felt forgotten about because he had to wait
for a long time for the doctor to come and attend to his

intravenous infusion. He waited $5\frac{1}{2}$ hours for the doctor to come and set up a drip. He felt neglected, but at the same time Ed defended the staff by emphasizing how busy the nurses and doctors were. That's why they left him unattended for so long:

"... as I was saying there were other things doing and all. I don't suppose they can be in two places at once. But you're not the only one, I expect there were others worse than I was like, that needed attending to".

The role of the hospital environment

It should be clear that just arriving in hospital and settling into the routines to await an uncertain future is a complicated and anxiety-provoking experience. The physical environment, the technology, the uniformed staff and the specialist language used by the staff are all influential and contribute to the feeling of crushing vulnerability that many, if not all, patients experience. In short:

When a patient is admitted to hospital, he finds himself in a strange environment and an alien culture. He is usually apprehensive, because he has a condition considered to be too serious to be treated in the doctor's office. The intensity of his apprehension increases with his uncertainty about what to expect in hospital. Much of what will happen in the hospital depends upon tests and procedures to be done there; for example, laboratory test results may indicate the need for an exploratory operation. Depending on what is found at operation, there may be a need for radical surgery, chemotherapy, or no treatment—possibly the difference between life and death. *Uncertainty reigns* (Leigh and Reiser, 1980, p. 281).

Patients as objects

The people interviewed during the study were at the mercy of the illness and the professional care system. The feeling of 'crushing vulnerability' was uppermost in their minds. The strange hospital environment was daunting. Hospital was not really seen as a helping sanctuary but a place of fear and anxiety from which there was no escape. Being treated like an object in hospital was a source of great anxiety. Some of the patients were ignored as people and their personal details were discussed in public handovers from shift to shift, whereas other patients commented on the positive effect of being treated like a person while in hospital because it helped to promote recovery and made them feel good. This distinction may be similar to the I–it and I–thou types of relationships described by the philosopher Martin Buber (1958). In an I–it relationship one person treats another person like an object or thing showing little regard for the other person's needs. The I–thou relationship, on the other hand, may be regarded as a meeting of equals—two people coming together and displaying a mutual respect and concern for each other's welfare. The I–thou type of relationship is especially valuable in counselling (Burnard, 1989).

In a discussion of the role of *existential advocacy* in the nurse–patient relationship, Gadow (1980) outlined an important distinction between the different modes of access that nurses and patients have to the patient's body as follows:

> Because patient and nurse have fundamentally different modes of access to the patient's body, and thus experience it in opposite ways, their understanding of it differs. The patient understands her body as a unique reality that cannot be expressed through types or generalisations. The nurse understands the patient's body as part of the world of objects, and therefore, most effectively approached through clinical categories. She is, of course, ultimately concerned with the patient as a unique human being, but she addresses the body's phenomena as instances of general types of phenomena...In their involvement with the patient's body, the patient is oriented toward uniqueness, the professional toward typification (p. 89).

In drawing attention to the impact of illness on a person's life, Van den Berg (1972b) ignored the medical concerns but observed the:

> ... changes in a sick person's existence, the changes in his life which suddenly confront a person when he finds himself ill (p. 17).

The anxiety and vulnerability associated with being treated as an 'object' was also captured by Van den Berg (1972b) as follows:

> One of the most painful experiences of the sickbed is to discover again and again that one has become an 'object'. The 'sick body' is a thing at the disposal of the doctor and the nurse far more than it is with the patient himself. To discuss him in his presence is more evidence to him that he has become an object (p. 97).

A similar type of experience has been described by Goffman (1968) as being treated like a non-person as follows:

> ... the wonderful brand of 'non-person treatment' found in the medical world, whereby the patient is greeted with what passes as civility, and said farewell to in the same fashion, with everything in between going on as if the patient weren't there as a social person at all, but only as a possession someone has left behind (p. 298).

Crushing vulnerability emphasizes each patient's need for sensitive nursing care. Inappropriate or tactless handling can have devastating consequences for the patient. Only one patient of the 10 interviewed here was openly critical of the general care he received. He was made to feel like an object not a person. He had little say in his overall management, he was ignored during the handovers, his personal details were discussed publicly by the staff and he had little contact with the trained staff. All these subtle and not so subtle actions made him feel like an object.

What can be done to improve the situation

Several things can be done to help patients cope with the situation. Nurses can learn to become more aware of the vulnerability that patients, probably all patients who are hospitalized, experience. It is very easy to become complacent about hospital and illness if you are working in a hospital environment all of the time. Some staff cope with the stress of hospital work by deliberately cutting off the human and emotional side of things. They tell students 'not to get involved' with patients and to 'keep a safe distance' from patients. Being cold and dispassionate will not help nurses to care for the person who is a vulnerable patient. Overfamiliarity with hospitals and illness should not prevent nurses from recognizing that each new patient is primarily a person.

Nurses can also make a point of *spending time with patients*. It is not possible to get a clear understanding of what that person is really experiencing unless you sit down and *listen*. This practice does 'take up time' from the workings of the organization, and spending time with patients is often frowned upon by some ward managers who are more concerned with the image of the ward. Taking time and listening to the patient is also risky emotionally. It is difficult to know what the patient might say or do or how he or she will react. The best way to learn how to cope with these uncertainties is to do it. With experience you will find yourself better able to cope with these situations and better able to care for another person.

Summary

The vulnerability of the patient's world was highlighted. Not all patients respond in the same way to illness and hospitalization, but clearly the theme 'crushing vulnerability' captures an important facet of the way in which people respond as patients in a hospital context. This vulnerability may be linked directly to the types of behaviour that hospitalized patients display. The next chapter explores some of the modes of self-presentation that these patients displayed.

Further reading

Brown, L. (1986) The experience of care: patient perspectives. *Topics in Clinical Nursing*, 8 (2), 56–62.

Elbeck, M.A. (1986) Client perceptions of nursing practice. *Nursing Papers*, 18 (2), 17–24.

Evers, H.K. (1986) Care of the elderly sick in the UK. In: S.J. Redfern (ed.) *Nursing Elderly People*. Churchill Livingstone, Edinburgh, pp. 293–310.

Forrest, D. (1989) The experience of caring. *Journal of Advanced Nursing*, 14, 815–823.

Kelly, M.P. (1992) Health promotion in primary care: taking account of the patient's point of view. *Journal of Advanced Nursing*, 17, 1291–1296.

Knight, M. and Field, D. (1981) Silent conspiracy: coping with dying cancer patients on acute surgical wards. *Journal of Advanced Nursing*, 6, 221–229.

Lucente, F.E. (1972) A study of hospitalization anxiety in 408 medical and surgical patients. *Psychosomatic Medicine*, 34 (4), 304–312.

Stimson, G.V. (1974) Obeying doctor's orders: a view from the other side. *Social Science and Medicine*, 8, 97–104.

Van den Berg, J.H. (1972) *The Psychology of the Sickbed*. Humanities Press, New York.

Chapter 5

Patients adopted a particular mode of self-presentation

Throughout our lives attempts are made, either directly or indirectly, to influence the way we think, feel and behave. Similarly, we spend much time in social interaction attempting to influence others to think, feel or act as we do. Indeed the continuance of any society demands a degree of *conformity* to social norms; society also demands people *comply* with requests and *obey* authority at times. However, people are not sheep, they do not blindly conform, comply or obey whenever the opportunity arises ... the individual is often placed in the conflicting situation of needing to maintain his or her own sense of identity and independence whilst at the same time being required or expected to conform, obey or comply with other people's wishes, prevailing norms, or standard. Failure to fall in with the 'crowd' may incur painful penalties ... failure to achieve and maintain a sense of identity may result in low self-esteem, low self-confidence and, in more extreme cases, depression and apathy (Pennington, 1986).

Introduction

In this chapter the different modes of self-presentation adopted by patients in hospital are examined. These modes of self-presentation helped patients to cope with the situations they had to face up to. The different modes of self-presentation are likely to be influenced by a wide range of factors including personality types, previous experience of hospital, the patient group, the nature of the illness and the level of family and social support available. In addition, the institution itself, the organizational culture and the ways the staff behave towards patients will also determine how the patients respond to their circumstances as a whole.

The social setting found in a hospital ward can place *demand characteristics* on the patient and his or her behaviour changes to fit in with what is required in that social situation. The demand characteristics have been described as 'aspects of any social situation providing tacit or implicit cues as to the behaviour expected' (Pennington, 1986, p. 12) and these have been found to influence people's behaviour in psychological experiments. Behaviour here refers to overt behaviour and attitudes.

Orne (1962) noted that the demand characteristics of the psychology experiment entails cooperating with the experimenter and giving the experimenter the type of data needed to run a successful experiment. The experiment requires that the 'subject' is a 'good subject'. The social world of the hospital can also work like a psychology laboratory to produce 'good' patients. Think of this theory when you read about the patients' modes of self-presentation that follow in this chapter. The organization and layout of the qualitative findings is identical to that in Chapter 4. The main theme—patients adopted a particular mode of self-presentation—is expanded with appropriate headings and subheadings.

PATIENTS ADOPTED A PARTICULAR MODE OF SELF-PRESENTATION

This is the second major theme to have emerged from the interviews with patients. To survive in the environment and protect their self-esteem, patients had to adapt to the hospital setting. They had to 'fit in' by whatever means were available to them. Several of the patients noted changes in their own behaviour that were linked to being ill and in hospital. They were able to recall and relate these to me during the interviews. They *adapted* themselves to cope. They adopted particular modes of self-presentation and the hospital environment contributed by placing certain demand characteristics on the patients. Assuming the roles appears to have been done consciously in some cases and without awareness in others. Here are some of the modes of presentation that were identified during the analysis of the interviews:

(a) Became sheepishly obedient
Some patients became very obedient. Florence did everything that the staff told her to do:

> "Maybe I'm a bit sheepish".

She looked to doctors, nurses and other professionals when things went wrong and she was uncertain about what she should do. She had 'blind faith' in the professionals who cared for and looked after her. James too was led by the needs of the staff. He always ensured that he gave staff the correct information. He did not want to waste the staff's time, and he did what was asked of him unquestioningly.

Tim, an extremely nervous patient, met with many medical students because of his complicated and medically interesting condition. It was not easy to be confronted by all of these powerful and professional people, and he was very nervous about all the attention he received. He did, however, put up with all the requests to be examined and probed because he felt he would be foolish to be awkward and uncooperative with the people who treated him. George made it easier for the staff to take blood and was very cooperative during investigations by removing his dressing gown and preparing himself patiently on his bed for the different investigators.

The interesting thing here is that the type of obedience that these patients displayed is more characteristic of children awaiting parental rewards than that expected of adults. Most people (adults) surely want to know *why* blood is sampled, *what* the treatments mean, *who* will perform the procedure and so on. These are very reasonable and sensible bits of information that any adult would want before he or she agrees to 'comply' and 'cooperate with' the medical and nursing staff. Clearly, these patients must have received some demand characteristics from the social situation. It may be that patients *model* themselves on other patients who have been in the ward for a longer time. The implicit and explicit messages about how to behave are likely to shape patient behaviours. It is possible that some patients do not wish to 'know' things about their operation or treatment and their views must also be respected. However, these individuals are more the exception than the rule: most people want to know what is happening to them even if this means hearing 'bad' news (Kent and Dalgleish, 1986).

(b) Conformed to the ritualistic practice

Another mode of self-presentation involved conforming to the ritualistic practices that staff performed. George, for example, felt that patients generally needed to abide by the ritualistic practice of the medicine round if the work was to get done in an effective and efficient manner. He was not allowed to collect his medicine from the medicine trolley but did collect his own tea from the tea trolley. George believed that regimentation was necessary for survival and so he was happy to be part of the regimented style of care that he was exposed to.

(c) Became unusually friendly and cheerful

In a hospital there is suffering, pain and death all around the patients and staff. Some patients get better and are discharged; others undergo a period of prolonged suffering and die. It is interesting to note how different patients coped with the anxieties and uncertainties that the hospital ward must have aroused. One strategy that appears on the face of it to be paradoxical is to adopt an unusually friendly and cheerful disposition. This strategy is usually warmly welcomed by the staff. Everybody likes a happy and friendly patient who cheers up the staff as well as other members of the patient group.

Several patients adopted a cheerfulness that was unfitting for the awful situations in which they found themselves. One tried to be liked by the staff and hoped the staff saw her as a cheery sort of person. As a result she hoped the staff enjoyed looking after her. However, she did not feel obliged to be cheerful, because Florence was by nature a cheerful sort of person and she hoped the staff did not mind looking after her. Other patients felt obliged to try to be cheerful. However, one long-stay patient, Martha, described her stay as being as happy as it could have been in the circumstances. She had a sense of resignation that she would just have to put up with the situation she was in if she was to recover. It was beyond her control to do anything about it.

(d) Provided a frank and honest account

One of the patients developed an attitude of openness and honesty with staff that meant they knew a great deal about him and his life while he knew very little about them. This imbalance of shared information would not really occur in other facets of a person's life, but in a hospital context this is a routine practice and the 'correct' thing to do. Through this imbalance the patients' vulnerability is heightened while the power and status of the professional carer is enhanced.

George made sure he answered the staff's questions honestly and told the truth about his excessive drinking:

> "They asked me and I told them the truth and helped in that way. That's all part of the system ... the set up. I mean it's

stupid to tell them one pint a day when I'm drinking fourteen.
But some people do these things''.

He weighed up the pros and cons of such self-disclosure. Not
to tell the whole truth could damage his chances of improvement and recovery through ineffective medical management of
his condition. To disclose information about his drinking
weakened his self-esteem and exposed him to the risk of being
sanctioned or ignored by the staff like an unpopular patient.
Medical conditions associated with drinking alcohol may be
attributed by the staff as being his own fault.

The psychologist Sidney Jourard (1964) suggests that 'self-
disclosure begets self-disclosure'. In other words, the more we
tell other people about ourselves the more they will tell us
about themselves. This may be true when we are at a party or
sharing a long train journey with a stranger, but in a hospital
the style of self-disclosure is usually one-sided. Patients are
there because they are ill and need help. They must disclose
things about themselves, sometimes of a very intimate and
personal nature, to enable the staff to do their work. That is fine
as far as the work is concerned, but psychologically that leaves
the patients in an underprivileged and weak position in the
social world of the ward.

(e) Helpful camaraderie amongst patients
Groups of total strangers with different levels of education,
socioeconomic backgrounds and cultures can be found on any
hospital ward. They have been thrown together by chance. One
factor brings them closer together—the experience of illness.
Through the time spent in hospital together, these people are
drawn closer both physically and psychologically. They need
the support of their relatives and the professional care staff.
Doctors and nurses do not spend a great deal of time with
patients and family members can only be with them for
specified and short visiting times. Patients often develop a

comradeship amongst themselves to help and support each
other.

They make a point of helping each other. Florence tried to
help other patients settle into the ward, although she did not see
herself as a 'goody-goody' person. Eileen was not desperately
ill or in need of a lot of physical care and found herself
spending her time completing meal cards for the elderly
patients and helping out generally at mealtimes. However, she
did not 'take over' the situation from the staff. She knew where
to draw the line and did not interfere with the work of the
organization. She only helped out so that the older patients
were not left alone and unable to eat by themselves. Staff
appreciated her help. Helping other patients was enjoyable and
Eileen wanted to help the staff in any way she could. Al
generally got on well with people. He made sure that he went
around the ward and talked to other patients during the day.
The patients on the ward became pals. There was a camaraderie between patients.

The enforced camaraderie in the hospital ward obviously
helps patients. It surely reduces boredom and helps to pass the
time. Much of the patients' day is spent 'waiting' for other
people to come to the ward and for investigations and routines
to be completed. Nurses need to think carefully about how
patients can be helped to cope with boredom in hospital. Not
all patients can find comradeship in the ward, especially those
in side wards or single rooms. Remember that televisions and
radios can become very boring after a short time. They lack the
spontaneity of human contact.

These small groups are also likely to help patients talk about
their illness, investigations, treatments and so on as a way of
dealing with anxiety. For the most part this small group activity
works well for many patients. Unfortunately, it can go wrong.
Some patients may become more anxious about their treatment
and care because of the things that other patients have told
them in an informal way. We need to be aware of this danger

and ensure that all of the people in our care are kept properly informed and up-to-date. Patients need time to voice their anxieties. Nurses need time to deal with these effectively. This aspect of care must be planned.

(f) Reluctant to ask questions

Although the patients' need for information about their illness and treatment was great, patients were generally reluctant to ask questions about their care and treatment. It would appear that patients were not encouraged to ask questions of the staff and this may be another demand characteristic that is part of the hospital culture. When patients did ask questions about aspects of their care, the staff used subtle tactics for letting the patients know that they should not ask such questions: they let the patient know how busy they were; gave the impression that the patient was being a nuisance; or provided incomplete answers to the patient's questions. These tactics had the effect of closing down any further communication between the patient and the nurse and ensured that a further detailed questioning did not occur.

This reluctance to ask questions is unhealthy. If we want patients to assume greater responsibility for their own health and well-being, to comply with health education instructions and become involved in decisions about their own medical management, we must actively encourage patients to ask us questions. There is a very large body of research that clearly demonstrates the positive effects of providing patients with information about their care. Well-informed patients require less analgesia, recover more quickly and comply more readily with health education advice (see for example Ley, 1988, 1989).

Needed to keep up-to-date

The issue of whether to ask questions and seek out information was important to several patients. Some patients refrained from

asking questions altogether, while others limited their questioning to the sort of questions that had a simple 'yes' or 'no'
answer. This meant that the questions did not make the staff
feel uneasy and lead into any tricky and emotional areas.
Patients were aware of their lack of knowledge. There was a lot
going on that James did not know about. On some wards
patients were better informed and not all patients needed to ask
questions. George had no need to ask many questions because
he was kept up-to-date with accurate information and pic-
tures—diagrams that displayed what was entailed in the
surgical procedure—and his questions were answered.

Did not want to bother the staff by asking questions
It was suggested that the staff must convey implicitly, and
sometimes explicitly, messages to patients about how to
behave in the ward. One way of ensuring that patients did not
ask searching questions was to give the impression of 'busy-
ness'. It is true that many wards are busy and understaffed, but
this is not so on all wards and at all times. There is, in the
hospital culture, a tacit obligation to 'look busy', and this
obviously was noted by some patients. Students too often
comment on this 'value' within the organizational culture on
returning from clinical placements.

The patients who took part in this study were not encouraged
to ask questions of the staff, although nobody actually told
James *not to ask questions*. However, Hugh was made to feel
like a nuisance for asking questions and this was particularly
marked when he asked the doctors. Tim did not want to bother
the staff by asking probing questions; he felt that staff could
not give an honest answer until the test results were known.
Tim felt confident that the staff would tell him if anything was
wrong. One of the patients became more confident and asked
questions of the staff, but this was in contrast to all the other
patients around him who did not ask questions because they
felt it was not right to bother the busy nurses. When questions

were asked the staff answered these as best they could in an open and honest fashion.

(g) Kept interpersonal encounters superficial

Another strategy that some patients used was to keep interpersonal encounters brief and superficial. James deliberately set limits on the contact he had with others in the ward group. He became part of a patient group, but even these encounters with other patients were limited. He did not talk at length about his illness and treatment. He kept the conversations focused on superficial things like the weather, sport and television. He made sure that more 'permanent relationships' were not established during his time in hospital, even though the relationships he did have made him feel cared for by the other people in the ward group. Close relationships with nurses were also not developed; indeed some patients preferred to keep their distance from the staff:

> "It's me. That's the way I am, that's the way I've lived. I'm an ex-headmaster, I've had to learn to draw lines".

George kept to himself and read; he did not go looking for conversations, but he talked constantly to his wife during the visiting time. Another patient, Ed, felt that the nurses did what they had to do and no more. They were not interested in, or supposed to get closer to, patients in hospital.

(h) Tried not to be a nuisance

Several patients mentioned how they tried not to be demanding or to bother the staff. They tried not to be a 'nuisance'. James kept out of the way especially when the staff were ill-tempered:

> "... they come on to a shift at seven in the morning after getting up at six and people can get up out of the wrong side of the bed. If you notice that, you know to keep your head down".

When Ed was recovering and preparing to be discharged, he just spent his time marching up and down the ward outside of his room. Martha, who spent nearly 2 months in hospital and who needed a lot of care after her surgery, suggested that 'not being a nuisance' meant that other patients got their fair share of care and attention from the staff. Martha did not feel guilty about asking for help generally, but sometimes she was *made to feel guilty* by the staff who let her know that other patients on the ward also needed looking after.

(i) Provided a sense of purpose for the carers

Patients are admitted to hospital because they need special care and treatment. They are in a very vulnerable position. Nevertheless, several patients felt that they were able to give something back to the staff who cared for them. Florence felt that she was able to provide the carers with a sense of achievement, while Zoe felt that seeing people get better helped nurses to do their work and provided them with a sense of purpose. Not everyone felt this way: Martha felt that she had very little to give back to the carers. She was at times totally dependent on them for everything.

(j) Showed deference and gratitude to the carers

In general, patients are very grateful for the care they receive. Al always displayed good manners and 'thanks' to the carers who looked after him. He really appreciated what was done for him. He always called the nurse 'nurse' and would not dare to call them by their first names. George wanted to give money to the NHS and felt many others would do the same.

(k) Admired the hard-working staff

There was much admiration for the work done by the staff for the patients in their care. Several patients expressed the view that nurses did not do the job 'just for money'. Zoe could not understand how the nurses did some of the 'awful jobs' that they had to do. However, she was very glad someone did it. She was incontinent a couple of times during her admission and the young students had to clean it up; she felt so sorry for them. Zoe also suggested that the nurses were 'dedicated'. George stressed the view that nursing was partly a vocation and a vocation was necessary for survival in this type of work. The younger nurses especially had 'the vocation'. Florence felt that it was possible to train nurses to care, but only if it was part of their personality make-up.

Self-presentation and survival in hospital

The crushing vulnerability that patients experience helps us to understand why patients display different modes of self-presentation in hospital. The vulnerable patients had to *survive* in the hospital environment by whatever means they could. They had to adjust to illness and hospitalization. They needed to be perceived by the staff as people 'worthy' of care by being vulnerable and in need of help. They also had to maintain their self-esteem. By fitting into the hospital environment and meeting the demand characteristics of the situation they could do this.

A number of strategies of self-presentation were used by the patients. Some became sheepishly obedient or conformed to the ritualistic practices of the ward. However, excessive compliance motivated by fear can be unhelpful and lead to what Ley (1988) called 'malignant compliance'. This is a form of good patient behaviour that can lead to a worsening in the patient's condition, e.g. patients who continue to take medication that has dangerous side-effects simply because the doctors told them to keep taking the medication until their next appointment.

Others became unusually cheerful and friendly in a situation that was terrifying and anxiety-provoking for the patients and probably for their relatives as well. These strategies of self-presentation are likely to be well received by the staff, and fit in well within the organizational culture. Cheerful, deferential and compliant patients are much more 'popular' than articulate, awkward and questioning patients (Stockwell, 1972). People who work in hospitals tend to take the environment and all its 'trappings' for granted. Patients, relatives and others unfamiliar with the setting see it as an alien place and are often struck by an uncertainty about how to fit in. Conforming to the implicit and explicit demands of the staff is a 'safe' mode of self-presentation.

Some patients slotted in by providing a frank and honest account of their home and life circumstances. They made no attempt to cover up aspects of their lives that they might do normally in other social situations. They 'confessed' to the professional staff. The friendly camaraderie amongst the patients themselves was also found in another study by Coser (1962). In these small groups patients had other people to talk to during the day and could exchange stories about their conditions, daily progress and things outside of the hospital. When it came to asking questions of the staff, however, patients were very reluctant. Coser (1962) also noted how new patients on a ward quickly learned 'what' to ask and 'what not' to ask, and 'who' to ask. It seems that the situation described by Coser is still a relevant and accurate account of how patients behave in hospital.

Ley (1988) argued that patients' reluctance to ask questions stemmed '...mainly from over-deferential attitudes towards doctors' (p. 16). Patients kept their interpersonal encounters superficial, filled with idle talk about the weather and so on. Patients were careful to ensure that they were not perceived by the staff to be a nuisance. They did not want to bother the staff or to alienate them. All these tactics helped them to cope with the anxiety about illness and the uncertainty associated with being in hospital. In another research study, Waterworth and

Luker (1990) emphasized the importance of 'toeing the line' as a patient.

Respectful admiration for the staff

Some patients felt that by being a patient in hospital they also provided a sense of purpose for the carers, because without patients there would be no nurses to look after them. Many patients showed admiration, deference and gratitude to the carers. It seemed almost to be an expectation of the role of being a patient to do so, and most patients fulfilled this requirement without hesitation. Showing admiration for the dedicated staff ensured that patients would be seen in a positive light by the staff. In a discussion of the social rules governing deference and demeanour, Goffman (1956) noted how the *expectations* of one group *confers an obligation* on another group to behave in certain ways. The nurses' expectations of conforming, compliant and uncomplaining patients may lead patients to behave in these expected ways. If the expectations are not met, then the staff have the power to ignore or sanction that person and ensure that all the other members of the caring team do likewise.

One patient in particular commented on the way he spoke to the nurses. He always addressed the nurses as 'nurse' even though he got to know particular nurses quite well during his stay in hospital. This had the effect of reinforcing the unequal status that separated the nurse and the patient. It was an overt mechanism for displaying deference to the staff. This nurse–patient relationship is obviously not one of equals because the carer seems to be giving all the time and receiving little in return. There is no 'reciprocal' relationship between the nurse and patient, although it seems likely that on occasions a close bond does develop between some patients and nurses. As a rule, however, the hospital setting does not facilitate this type of close and mutual relationship. In addition, the deferential mode of presentation adopted by many patients may well serve as a means of legitimizing the professional, caring and powerful role of the nurse.

It was also interesting how staff used the patients' first names to address them even though many of the patients in their care were older and more senior than the nurses. This is another interaction strategy that helps to empower the staff and increase their status over the patients. However, some of the patients admitted that they liked being called by their first names because it made them feel human, even if it meant being an extremely vulnerable human. The nurses were also allowed to touch patients and come into very close contact with them to perform nursing tasks such as washing. This ability was never questioned by patients.

The demeanour of both patients and staff (Goffman, 1956) also played a role in determining the behaviour of nurses and patients. The patients were dressed in night attire, although only one or two of them needed to be at the time of the interviews. The nurses were dressed in their uniforms, with coloured epaulettes, pens, notebooks and so on, all of which instantly displayed their grade and level of expertise to patients and visitors to the ward. The demeanour of the patients and nurses helped to reinforce the differences in status and position in the hospital. The balance of power was very one-sided.

What can be done to improve the situation

Clearly if nurses are to treat patients as people they need to be aware of the subtle and not so subtle demands that are placed on them at a time of tremendous personal vulnerability. Several other sources lend support for the rich picture that has emerged here (see for example Broome, 1989; Fallowfield, 1991; Toombs, 1992; Audit Commission, 1993). If the experiences of the patients involved in this study are typical, then the need for more sensitive nursing care of patients is obvious. Nurses can help to bring about changes in their own work style and consequently changes in the way the organization works by focusing on some of the following areas.

Observe patients very carefully taking note of both verbal and non-verbal behaviour and the particular context in which these observations are made. Remember to check your observations with those of other members of staff to ensure 'objectivity'. It is easy to make errors of attribution and these may influence the clinical judgements that staff make about patients. Nurses can also ask the patient if their interpretation and/or understanding of the patient is correct. This particular strategy may open up the possibility of further discussion with the patient and help nurses to get a more detailed picture of what the patient is thinking and feeling. Many qualitative researchers ask their informants if their interpretations are correct. They do this to ensure that they have an accurate representation of what informants said and meant during interviews. Practising nurses need to do likewise. Good clinical assessments and judgements can only be made after sufficient information about patients has been gathered and checked for accuracy.

It was noted in Chapter 3 that people have a tendency to make causal attributions to explain why others react as they do. Try to avoid making overelaborate theories to explain patients' behaviour and attitudes. Develop your own self-awareness by monitoring some of the attributions you make about patients and their families. This may take time and a great deal of personal honesty, but the end result will be well worth the effort made. It is all too easy just to fit in with what the ward team thinks and act accordingly. Such actions and attitudes may be of little use to the person/patient being cared for and who needs help and support.

Some patients come into hospital and assume the sick role in textbook fashion. Try to encourage patients who become overdependent to take responsibility for themselves. This has to be done tactfully and sensitively. Nurses may have to withdraw support gradually over time as patients assume greater responsibility for themselves. This is particularly important in the care of the long-term patient. Involve patients in decisions about their care. Keep them informed and give appropriate and understandable information. Check that they have *understood* what the nurse has said by asking them to explain it in their own words. Give them time to think about the issues raised. Explain clearly what these patients need to do to become more independent. Draw up goals for the patient with the patient's consent. It is sometimes very difficult to identify an overdependent patient. The best way of ensuring that your assessment is accurate is by working closely with the patient and talking through the programme of planned nursing care. This process helps the nurse to find out what the patient can do independently and when he or she may need assistance.

Learn to *evaluate nursing openly and honestly*. Develop a supportive network with trusting colleagues and evaluate each other's performance as a nurse. It takes time, patience and honesty to develop good working relationships like this. It is also very threatening to do this in the beginning, but with experience it is possible to learn through self-awareness and the end product of this learning will be more effective and high-quality care for patients.

Finally, learn to accept your privileged position as a nurse, but do not misuse the power that goes along with this role. Accept this important role with humility. Ask yourself how you would feel if the patient was *your* mother, husband or child? Would you be happy with the style of care given? Remember too that each patient is *someone's* mother, father, sister, brother, friend or spouse.

Summary

In this chapter the second major theme that characterized the patients' point of view was examined. It was noted how patients adopted particular modes of self-presentation, which in themselves seemed immature and maladaptive, but in the hospital setting seemed to be very appropriate responses to the expectations that were placed on them by staff and the organizational culture generally. The issue of professional power emerged as an important element in determining how staff behave with patients and consequently as a means of getting patients to behave in ways that minimize the emotional burden and workload on staff.

Further reading

Audit Commission (1992) *Making Time for Patients. A Handbook for Ward Sisters*. HMSO, London.

Audit Commission (1993) *What Seems to be the Matter. Communication Between Hospitals and Patients*. HMSO, London.

Evers, H. (1981) Care or custody? The experiences of women patients in long-stay geriatric wards. In: B. Hutter and U. William (eds) *Controlling Women: The Normal and the Deviant*. Croom Helm, London.

Hugman, R. (1991) *Power in Caring Professions*. Macmillan, London.

Illich, I. (1975) *Medical Nemesis: The Expropriation of Health*. Calder and Boyars, London.

Jeffrey, R. (1979) Normal rubbish: deviant patients in casualty departments. *Sociology of Health and Illness*, 1 (1), 90–107.

Jourard, S. (1964) *The Transparent Self*. Van Nostrand, Princeton, New Jersey.

Mittler, P. (1979) *People Not Patients*. Methuen, London.

Rose, S. and Black, B. (1985) *Advocacy and Empowerment: Mental Health Care in the Community*. Routledge and Kegan Paul, London.

Wolinsky, F.D. and Wolinsky, S.R. (1981) Expecting sick role legitimation and getting it. *Journal of Health and Social Behaviour*, 22 (3), 229–242.

Chapter 6

Patients evaluated the services provided in hospital

One of the problems of trying to evaluate good practice in mental health services is the lack of specific aims and objectives associated with current health policy. One can safely say that there is general consensus about moving from a system of warehousing people in large Victorian asylums to 'care in the community'. However, over and above this global objective, there appear to be few agreed principles about the look of a post institutional world. The present philosophy underlying mental health planning seems *ad hoc* rather than coherent; full of good intentions but not fully worked out (Rogers *et al.*, 1993).

Introduction

In this chapter the third major theme uncovered during the analysis of the patient interviews is examined. It deals with the ways in which patients *evaluate* the care they receive. As part of the modes of self-presentation considered in the previous chapter, it could be anticipated that patients evaluate the care that they received in a very positive light. To do otherwise suggests that they have not fully complied with the expected 'good patient' role that is part of the hospital culture.

Indeed, it is probably fair to say that when patients are asked to evaluate the care and treatment they have received in a *general way*, they usually say very positive things about the hospital and the staff. In this chapter the phenomenological approach used in the study permitted the patients to express very positive comments about the care they received, but at the same time, very specific deficiencies were also identified by individual patients. These have been described and some tentative interpretations have been offered. The organization and layout of the chapter follows the previous two chapters.

PATIENTS EVALUATED THE HOSPITAL SERVICES

The routine hospital facilities and resources and the manner in which staff interacted with the patients was evaluated by the patients during the time spent in hospital. Generally these evaluations were positive, but there were instances where patients were overtly critical of the staff and the organization. It is possible that the resources, the service and the people involved in delivering day-to-day care became the living *symbols of a caring service* as all the patients declared openly that they did not get close to any of the nursing staff throughout the time spent in hospital. This was surprising. As nurses, we constantly affirm the importance of getting to know each individual patient well as the foundation for making nursing care plans. Yet here, the analysis of the personal experiences of 10 patients interviewed about their care in hospital suggested that these patients did not get to know any of the staff well. They did, however, make evaluations about their care.

(a) General level of satisfaction with the caring staff
There was a general level of satisfaction with the care received and many patients genuinely appreciated what was done for them. As consumers, they were satisfied with the level of care. The staff were perceived to be very caring and good, but some patients commented that none of the nurses were 'especially caring'—they just did what they were paid to do and no more. The technical facets of the nurses' role were primary. Ed felt

that hospital was the best place for him; staying at home with nobody to look after him was not a good idea. In other hospitals James found that the staff were not so caring, but in this hospital the staff were excellent. Florence felt good knowing that the staff were 'doing their best' for her.

Limited but satisfactory level of nursing care
The level of contact between the professional carers and the patients did appear to be very limited. Limited contact with consultants may be expected because they may have several hospitals to 'cover', and from more junior doctors to a lesser extent. As far as nurses are concerned this is very surprising. Nurses usually pride themselves on the fact that they are constantly available for patients. While doctors are 'on call', nurses are in fact the only group directly available for 24 hours of the day.

Not every patient had a lot of nursing attention; some did not have any 'real' nursing (basic/physical nursing care), only 'tests' such as chest X-rays, blood and urine investigations. These patients were described by the staff as 'self-caring' and received only a very limited amount of nursing care. On the surgical ward this usually entailed pre-operative preparation. James was very happy with all the attention he received, from the consultant down to the nurses. Some of the patients maintained that 'staff let the patients know they were there for them if they really needed them'. Because some of the patients did not need a lot of physical care, the contact with the nurses was limited to the times when the nurses had to perform some task or observation that was concluded quickly.

The limited contact between the nurses and some of the patients could mean that the psychological care of patients was lacking in this context. The need for physical care often presents the nurse with an opportunity for 'talking' to the patient and exploring that patient's personal view of the world. Unless nurses make a very deliberate attempt to care for the 'self-caring' patient psychologically, then these individuals will not be cared for adequately. This idea is discussed in more depth later.

High levels of nursing care needed
Other patients needed lots of physical care. Zoe, for example, needed to be helped in and out of the bath initially and then helped to walk as part of her rehabilitation and preparation for discharge. Gradually she became more independent and needed less and less help from the nurses. There was evidence here that the staff provided very thoughtful nursing and tried to prevent overdependence. In the beginning the nurses had to do everything for Zoe. As time passed they brought the equipment to Zoe and let her do her own dressing as soon as it was feasible for her to do so. Another patient, Tim, spent 9 weeks in four different hospitals undergoing a series of tests and different types of treatment for his complicated condition. He felt that he was treated the same in all of the hospitals he spent time in.

(b) Staff were friendly but diplomatic
Although the contact between patients and nursing staff was limited, several patients commented on the positive effect of having 'friendly' staff around them in the ward. Nobody was 'rude' to Tim in hospital. The friendly staff made some patients feel more at home. The informal and friendly atmosphere was helpful to patients and the staff. It made everybody feel more positive and optimistic. The nurses were always smiling. Zoe also commented on the friendliness of the staff, but she noted how 'careful' and 'diplomatic' the staff were when talking about her condition:

> "Well, they're very pleasant, they're very careful what they tell you. I asked when I will get better, what caused it and so on. But they're always very very careful and very diplomatic what they say …".

(c) Nurses asked what the patients needed

The approach of the staff was helpful and noted by several patients. Martha was confined to bed for some time and without frequent visitors. She found that most of the nurses asked if she needed washing or shopping done. Nurses who paid attention to detail were able to identify specific patient needs. One young student nurse took Martha's dressing gown home with her overnight and washed it for her. Some nurses also brought in magazines for her to look at to help pass the time and alleviate boredom.

(d) Felt safe and trusted the nurses

Martha was very dependent because of the major surgery she had. The nurses had to do a lot for her and she trusted the nurses and felt at ease with them. She felt safe because they held her firmly when she had to get into the bath, though some nurses made her feel safer than others.

(e) Technical competence was appreciated

Many patients praised the skill and expertise that characterized the nurses' performance. Injections were administered competently and sensitively, and blood samples were taken speedily and without inflicting unnecessary discomfort. Staff also ensured medicines were given on time. Tim noted how the steroid medications were reduced gradually to reduce any risks to him. Zoe commented that the experienced nurses were good at handling drips and dressings and so on, though this was not always true of less experienced nurses. It was clear that patients evaluated the performance of the staff and recognized more competent behaviour.

The nurses had to wash Ed and clean up any mess that he made, but he still developed a pressure sore on his back because he was left in one position for so long. The sore healed eventually by the nurses turning Ed regularly and encouraging him to be more mobile. They got him to walk up and down the corridor. The willingness with which help was given impressed Al greatly, and the way the staff checked his wound and dressed it every day reassured him that he was in good hands. Eileen also appreciated the speed with which she was admitted to hospital; she was glad to be in hospital, and stayed for 5 days. The rapid response of the professional team was reassuring. Zoe was also very ill on admission and appreciated being looked after by competent staff.

Nurses made constant checks on the patients and responded promptly when someone rang a call bell. The nurses were perceived by the patients to be 'always on their toes' and 'earned their money'. Ed had to use the call bell a couple of times when he was confined to bed and the staff always responded promptly.

(f) The approach of the staff was sensitive and calming
The nurses' ability to calm Tim, a very anxious patient, without resorting to the use of minor tranquillizers was important. Tim believed that the nurses did not know he had cancer. When Al came into hospital he was very apprehensive, but the staff quickly dispelled any fears that he had. Nurses also recognized the importance of being 'approachable' in a caring role (Morrison, 1991).

Watched the carers in action from a distance
In a hospital setting patients become observers of the way in which the staff manage other patients. George watched the nurses and doctors in action from a distance. He could not help overhearing things as the nurses calmed a very frightened patient. The caring nurses just sat with the frightened patient and they could not have done more for him. They quickly arranged for a social worker to help the patient's wife who was alone and disabled. They instilled confidence into the patient who was acutely ill and very frightened. The doctors and nurses were observed helping other upset and emotional patients.

Aware that the nurses understood her loneliness

When Martha's husband came to visit her at the weekend the nurses gave her husband a spare meal so that he could stay with her and not have to go down to the canteen some distance from the ward. The nurses knew he had to travel a long distance to be with her and in a few short hours he would have to travel 'up north' again by train to look after Martha's sick mother. This 'bending of the rules' by the nurses had a big impact on the way Martha perceived the nursing staff. She knew now that they recognized how lonely and vulnerable she felt and they tried to ensure that she and her husband had as much time together as possible.

(g) The accommodation and hotel services were reasonable

Several patients mentioned the importance of accommodation and hotel services during their stay in hospital. These aspects of their experience of being cared for are important for many patients. In general, the quality of the food was good, and the bed linen was changed daily. However, one patient noted that the china was cracked and ought to have been replaced. Zoe found the hospital clean and the atmosphere caring. At times the ward was short of staff, particularly at weekends, and patients noted a difference when this was so.

(h) The devoted students were constantly available

The student nurses were singled out by several patients for their attentive care and devotion. The younger nurses were very good and always available. One student introduced Florence to other patients on the ward soon after she was admitted and she felt much happier as a result. None of the patients objected to the fact that they were looked after mainly by student nurses rather than trained and more experienced nurses, because these young nurses had to gain experience to fulfil their training requirements. The 'constant availability' of the students was very notable and appreciated by patients.

The students took time and talked

Several patients referred to the contact they had with students. Students spent more time with the patients and got to know them better than the qualified staff; they were more caring. Some of the experienced students were very used to talking with patients and were very good at it. The students took time to talk to patients and shared 'a bit of their lives'—they did not simply collect information from the patients and give nothing back in return. Martha's relationship with the students was on a 'personal' and 'professional' footing because she spent such a long time in hospital, whereas most of the other patients in the ward were discharged much more rapidly.

The students listened and tried to answer questions

Talking to the students helped to keep Hugh's spirits up because they were very helpful. They 'listened' attentively to Hugh and tried to get answers to his questions from more senior members of staff when they could not answer his queries themselves. On one or two occasions, nurses tried to answer questions beyond their experience and knowledge, but Hugh knew when they did this. The students were also able to use a range of approaches when they talked to him—they were skilled at interacting because some of the general students had undergone psychiatric nurse training previously and this meant that they were more skilled interpersonally.

Appreciated the students who stayed late

Martha needed lots of physical care because she could not move much after the extensive surgery. She really appreciated when one of the students stayed on late to complete her care even though her shift had finished and other members of staff had gone home. The student did not want the new night shift to come in before she has finished settling Martha down for the night. This attention to detail was very notable.

Students went around with the doctors
Not all the patients were particularly appreciative of the students approach. Ed, who had little contact with students, noted how the students went around with the doctors. It was just as he had expected it to be in hospital. In general, the staff tended to ignore him.

(i) Helped to get through the miserable nights
The nights were mentioned by several patients as being difficult and unsettling. Zoe found the nights to be particularly hard because she could not sleep very well and became tired, miserable and fidgety. She found it upsetting to be woken up so early in the morning when she wanted a lie-in, but she had to fit in with the ward routine. Several patients commented that other patients coughing at night disrupted their sleep. However, several patients found the night staff to be particularly helpful because they made tea during the night to help patients sleep, just as they would do at home. Zoe found that the night nurses were genuinely interested and skilled in making her comfortable. The night staff were also pleased to see Zoe and asked how she was 'getting on' after they returned from their nights off. When they redressed her wound the night staff told her how well it was healing. They reassured her about her progress.

(j) Did not get to know nurses well
It is often claimed that the relationship between patients and nurses is the foundation for providing good nursing care. However, it was notable that, on the whole, patients did not get to know any of the nurses well. Contact between patients and nurses was often limited to tablet time. Nevertheless, some patients did not see a need to get to know the nurses well. They just wanted to be looked after by competent staff who treated them like 'people'—nothing more, nothing less. Patients did see a lot more of the students and unqualified nursing staff

because they came round regularly to do the observations (temperature, pulse, respiration and blood pressure), the washes and helped at meal times.

The level of interaction between nurses and patients presents the professional nurse with a dilemma. On the one hand the nurse must spend some time getting to know the patient in order to make an accurate clinical assessment of the patient's needs. The depth of such a relationship is difficult to specify. On the other hand many patients simply want to have their treatment and be looked after by competent staff and then go home feeling better. They do not want to develop close relationships with nurses and doctors. The skill is to be able to respond to the individual patient's needs, but it is difficult to achieve the right balance between these two extremes.

Minimal contact with qualified staff
Unlike the student group, the trained nurses spent even less time interacting with the patients. Hugh did not even speak to the ward sister at any time during his admission. He was very surprised that the qualified staff had so little time for him and the other patients. This was not the case on other wards where he had been a patient—there the staff made time for patients. The lack of contact with trained staff made a big difference to the patients' day. One of the patients observed how on one ward the qualified staff *found* things for the students to do if they saw them talking to patients or sitting down at the patient's bedside. Talking to patients was not 'the done thing'.

Superficial contact with nurses
When contact was established with the trained nursing staff it tended to have a superficial quality. George just passed the time of day with staff by talking about the weather, television, the most recent news items and so on. Some interactions with patients were limited to the nurse asking a patient to get off his

bed so that it could be made up and little else. One patient, Ed, felt that he did not get to know any of the nurses well; they did not mean a thing to him. The nurses did not talk to him except when they 'worked on him' to perform some procedure or administer medicines. In the end, he did not want them to talk to him and was content to remain alone during his stay on the ward.

The staff were awfully busy

Patients generally perceived the staff as being 'too busy' to talk to them or that other more serious patients needed attention more urgently. Eileen commented on the excellent staff nurse who was just too busy with all the other patients and did not have any spare time to spend with her. Several patients commented that the nurses were too busy and did not have time to talk:

> "The nurses didn't talk about the operation because they're awfully busy, they'll talk to you—yes. 'How are you today? How's your wound? Lets have a look at it, that's fine that's coming on nicely'. That sort of thing. But I mean they are awfully busy and there is a lot of physical work attached . . .''.

It was suggested that the really ill patients needed lots of attention and rest and the staff had to get on with their difficult work. It was also suggested that staff movements (shift patterns, staff reallocations and students' placements) were responsible for the lack of time available to the patients. Other patients were not bothered by staff movements and accepted the lack of interaction with the staff as a feature of the system of hospital care. Another patient felt that some staff *gave the impression* of being understaffed, while others were always relaxed and ensured that patients were well cared for no matter what pressure they were under. Students too have often commented on the 'impression management' that forms part of the hospital culture where 'being busy' is vital.

(k) Nothing was too much trouble

The attitude of the caring nurses was captured by several patients in this subtheme. Zoe felt that the staff were genuinely very busy, but they still gave the impression that 'nothing was too much trouble' for these busy staff. They put themselves out for her; they got the phone for her on many occasions and placed it beside her bed so that she could phone home. However, Zoe did not like asking for the phone because it really 'had nothing to do with her medical care and treatment'—it was a personal thing. Again this attention to apparently insignificant details can make a huge difference to the quality of care that many patients experience. On another occasion the staff got her iced water when it was very hot outside and the ward temperature was oppressive. They gave her everything they could within reason. Al too felt able to ask the staff for anything because nothing was too much trouble for the staff.

(l) No front—just genuine nurses

Tim commented that there was no 'front' to the nurses' attitude; they always displayed a concern 'for his well-being' and it was a genuine concern. An example of the genuine response of the staff was given when Tim described how the ward sister and the staff nurse on the ward cried when they found out he had cancer. Tim was very moved by their emotional response. It made him feel emotional too, but it was also comforting to know how these nurses felt about him and that they worried about him and what would happen to him ultimately. Hugh described the approach of the students as genuine and not patronizing—the qualified nurses were different.

(m) Displayed a caring attitude in their work

The nurses had time for the personal touch that was a crucial aspect of caring for George; they had what he described as a 'caring attitude' and it showed in the way they looked after the patients on the ward. There was no other way to describe how the nurses were; the phrase 'caring attitude' seemed to capture the nurses' disposition nicely for George.

(n) The doctors were approachable

Some doctors too were singled out for comment; the doctors were 'good and introduced themselves' to the patients when they came to the bedside. This made them more human and less frightening. The doctors allowed Florence to ask questions and she felt more confident when she did; she knew what was happening and what to expect in the coming days. Another patient openly expressed the view that the doctors and the treatment were 'exceptional'.

(o) Key criticisms of the staff

While many positive comments about the hospital and the staff were made during the interviews, several important criticisms also emerged that highlighted the need for staff to listen carefully to what patients have to say in order to evaluate nursing and medical care from the patients' perspective. This is an important step in meeting the needs of consumers and forms a starting point for continuous monitoring of nursing and medical care and for developing practices.

Rude staff

The importance of good manners was highlighted. George commented on the rude tea ladies, one of whom 'almost threw the tea' at him, and about the auxiliary nurse who was particularly rude. Another patient, Zoe, had an upsetting argument with a rude receptionist about her special diet and she became very upset and angry about the whole incident, which could easily have been avoided. She was so angry about the way she was treated that she felt like 'hitting' the reception-ist. The nurses were, however, very soothing and helped to

calm Zoe down after the incident with the receptionist. They
supported her, but they did not speak to the receptionist who
was at fault and ask her to apologize. These types of interpersonal incident can be very upsetting for patients, especially at a
time of anxious uncertainty. Support staff as well as nursing
staff need to be aware of this. Many upsetting incidents could
be avoided with a little thought and sensitivity.

Hurried approach of the nurses provoked anxiety
Martha needed extensive nursing care after her operations and
she did not like it when the nurses were 'in a rush'—especially
when she was in pain. Being rushed made her feel 'on edge' and
the nurses tended to 'dash through their work' when they were
short of staff. Zoe needed regular baths, and noticed that the
busy auxiliaries were constantly trying to get her into the bath in
a 'hurried' fashion. She just slotted into the regime that was
planned and organized by the auxiliaries because she had no say
in such matters. There wasn't much she could do to change
things; she just had to accept things the way they were and fit in
with the work routine. To do otherwise might lead to conflict.

Kept in the dark
Some patients felt that they were not given enough information
about their care and treatment. There was a general lack of
information on some wards, and sometimes patients had to ask
what their tablets were for. As mentioned earlier, to do this
runs the risk of being perceived by the staff as a 'complaining'
or 'bad' patient, but not knowing what the tablets are for may
lessen their importance in the patients' eyes. Hugh did not like
to take the tablets unless he knew exactly what they were for.
Several patients were not told why certain things were done
and that approach seemed 'normal' and routine:

  "... there's a definite lack of information. They do things but
  you don't know why half of the time".

It was even suggested by one of the patients that the staff in the hospital were 'trained to keep people in the dark' in a rather conspiratorial manner. The blame for not informing patients was placed firmly with the doctors and nurses by the patients who felt let down by the lack of information. The nurses and doctors were seen as the people responsible for telling people about illness, treatment, investigations and management. It may well be that staff need additional training in *how* to give information effectively by employing some principles from the psychology of memory such as primacy and recency, organization of information and reducing jargon (Ley, 1988).

Boredom

Although hospital wards are often very busy places, they may be very boring places for patients who are not acutely ill. Hospital became boring for Zoe after a while; she needed more things to do, but there were no activities organized on the ward. Once the staff did their essential 'preparation' on Zoe she was then left to 'entertain' herself by whatever means she could. This meant that she and most of the other patients were left in a strange environment within an alien hospital culture to 'wait' and think about what might happen to them. When Zoe became depressed in hospital she began to think about the mistakes she had made in her past life and just now she did not want to have time to think because it only made her feel more anxious and worried. She tried to talk to other patients to occupy herself, but she would have liked the staff to spend more time with her and just talk.

Poor nursing practice

One of the patients observed what she described as poor nursing practice. Eileen watched the nurses at mealtimes and noted how they gave the elderly patients far too much food in her view. Many of the older patients ate very slowly, some did not have their dentures in place during the meals and many could not eat the large portions of food that were supplied daily. Much of the food was wasted on the ward. Eileen was mobile and she took it upon herself to fill in the meal cards for the elderly patients who were unable to do this for themselves. She ordered smaller portions on the meal cards without consulting the nurses, who had not seen the need to do this.

This is a rather minor point, but it did highlight the need for the staff to pay greater attention to the needs of particular patients on the ward. The individual patients who were unable to eat the large portions or who did not have dentures surely appreciated Eileen's initiative, but this was something that the nurses ought to have seen to.

Service appraisal

It was difficult to see how the patients could have been critical of a system that, along with serious illness, made them so vulnerable and dependent. Their attention was focused on things that may seem unimportant to the staff. The friendliness of the staff was significant to patients. That the staff bothered to ask patients what they needed and the ability to make the patients feel safe influenced their opinions greatly. The technical competence of the staff in giving injections and other procedures was also much appreciated. The approach of the staff was sensitive and calming. All of these issues are relatively simple and straightforward elements of the nurses' daily work and contributed to the positive perceptions of the patients. It was clear that many members of staff were good at the job of caring for patients.

Symbolic hotel services

One important aspect of the experience of being cared for that tends to dominate patients' lives in hospital is the way they are looked after and the quality of the care they receive in hospital.

Rempusheski *et al.* (1988) suggested that the routine 'services' greatly influence perceptions of care that patients develop and the expressed level of satisfaction with those services. Doctors often achieved the status of 'heroes' and nurses were seen as 'dedicated and extremely hard working if underpaid individuals'. In this study, patients were generally satisfied with the care that they received, although some very pointed criticisms were mentioned and these tended to be things that could so easily have been put right with some careful planning and perhaps additional training.

Another aspect of the service that was appraised was the standard of hotel services offered to the patient. The accommodation and hotel services provided in hospital are not often considered by the staff as important. Indeed, in some units nurses have absolutely nothing to do with the provision of meals and drinks for patients and have little say in the quality of these services provided to their patients. There was evidence that some nurses pay little or no attention to patients' dietary intake. While this may seem reasonable to some because of changes in the way hotel services are delivered, it ignores the importance the patients place on these 'hotel' facilities. Having clean bed linen, or a clean and uncracked cup to drink out of, have symbolic meaning for the patients. They may convey to the patient a message that he or she is a *person worthy of care*, and not an object.

The patients interviewed here were well satisfied with the hotel services they received, and therefore nursing and medical staff and indeed other supportive colleagues can be generally pleased with the standard of care they provided for these patients. The student nurses and the night staff were singled out for praise, but the qualified and more senior nursing staff may need to think carefully about their role. Are they providers of direct patient care or managers of such services? The trained staff were generally perceived by patients as being too busy. This finding supports the general tendency for much of the basic nursing to be undertaken by the learners in particular or untrained staff (Knight and Field, 1981; Robinson *et al.*, 1989). This item will be discussed in more detail later on.

The apparently insignificant aspects of care in hospital, the attention to the sorts of detail that let the patients know they are appreciated and understood, should not be overlooked by professional carers. For patients they are important, at least in terms of their psychological well-being, and they are likely to influence their satisfaction with the quality of care received. These aspects of care may not rank as importantly as life-saving surgery, but to patients who come into hospital they are nevertheless very important. Many of these elements of the service can be easily monitored and high standards maintained. If nurses appreciate the significance of these facets of care, they can take account of them when monitoring and evaluating the service they provide for patients.

Why are patients so uncritical of the care they receive?

It was interesting that any criticism of the system emerged at all. Typically, patients are very reluctant to voice any criticism of the staff to anyone remotely involved in the system. This may be the result of an implicit rule of being a vulnerable patient—never criticise—because criticism is likely to lead to patients being labelled 'good' or 'bad' (Lorber, 1975; Kelly and May, 1982) or unpopular (Stockwell, 1972) and treated accordingly.

There are several possible reasons why these patients were not more critical of the care received. Most patients have very little 'status' in the social environment of the hospital. Many patients do not feel that they have any influence or control over what happens to them. They are not involved in decisions about their care. They passively accept things as they are, which may be an important part of the patient role that is entered into once the person becomes a patient. It is true that some patients do complain while in hospital, but others raise official complaints following discharge from hospital. It is notable that most of the official complaints about hospital highlight 'poor communication' as the major source of patient dissatisfaction. It is also notable that the number of official complaints about care has increased rapidly in recent years (Audit Commission, 1993).

In addition, to complain about your care to those who are looking after you will not endear you to the professional carers, who are 'human' too—nobody likes to be criticized. Patients are dependent on others for so much. To complain about any aspect of care is to run the risk of alienating those whose job is to care in a particular hospital setting. Moreover, staff may send 'messages' that it is 'not the done thing' to complain about them as a type of social 'demand characteristic'.

Another potential reason why patients were not outspoken was mentioned by Nehring and Geach (1973), who suggested that fear of reprisals from staff inhibits patients from expressing negative comments about the standards of care they receive:

> Most essential, it seems to us, is that we not ignore our most valuable source of information about our practice—our patients. We owe it not only to ourselves as professionals but also to the patients as consumers to devise means whereby their views can be ... put to use in planning, carrying out, evaluating, and researching our care ... It did not seem to strike the patients as forcibly as it struck us that there was a discrepancy between their idealised vision of nurses as dedicated professionals who would be there when *really* needed, and the other picture, also verbalised, of nurses who might withhold their services if one made a nuisance of oneself (Nehring and Geach, 1973, pp. 319–321).

The attitude of the staff may be crucially important here. If staff give these sorts of messages to patients to ensure that they conform to the expected norms of being a patient, then we should ask ourselves *why* this is so. The nurses' job is to reduce the effects of anxiety not to heighten it. Perhaps this is more evidence to support the hidden desire for 'power' over others that may be an inevitable facet of professional development in nursing. If this is a reasonable interpretation then we must be very clear about how we want to develop—do nurses want a professional helping role that actively promotes patients' independence or do they want a professional helping role that keeps patients in a state of powerlessness?

What can be done to improve the situation

The points mentioned in the last chapter will also apply here, but some additional pointers could be considered. Nurses should try not to overlook the importance of the 'apparently insignificant' aspects of the patient's situation. They need to pay attention to the 'hotel' services and satisfy themselves that these are as good as they ought to be. The small details can mean a lot to patients and can let patients know that you as a nurse understand what they may be going through and care about them.

There is a need to evaluate care and involve patients in those evaluations wherever possible. These evaluations must be open to constructive criticisms made by patients and other health-care colleagues. Practitioners could go to the library and find some evaluation questionnaires that could be used in their clinical areas. A team approach will work best here. Many evaluation instruments have been developed by researchers and these can help you to collect appropriate information for a fuller and more long-term evaluation of your own nursing unit.

Try to become familiar with the local complaints procedure and make sure that patients have easy access to it. Try to develop an 'open' atmosphere on the ward where colleagues and indeed patients can express their views honestly. Be prepared to listen to the views of others and take time to evaluate them. Try not to become defensive. If a patient makes an informal complaint about his or her care, investigate it and let the patient know what has been done. Tell patients about the outcomes of their complaints. Finally, do not be afraid to admit that sometimes you may get it wrong. Don't be arrogant.

Summary

Patients' evaluation of the care they received in hospital was examined. In general these evaluations were positive, but the phenomenological approach used in the study helped to identify many further details about the patients' experiences, and some of these highlighted important criticisms of the staff in the hospital and the care that the patients received. The evaluations were considered in the light of the patients' vulnerable and dependent position in the hospital system.

Further reading

Brandon, D. (1981) *Voices of Experience*. MIND, London.

Brechin, A. and Walmsley, J. (1989) *Making Connections. Reflecting on the Lives and Experiences of People with Learning Difficulties*. Hodder & Stoughton, London.

Downie, R.S. and Calman, K.C. (1987) *Healthy Respect. Ethics in Health Care*. Faber and Faber, London.

Fallowfield, L. (1990) *The Quality of Life. The Missing Measurement in Health Care*. Souvenir Press, London.

Holmes, C.A. (1989) Health care and the quality of life: a review. *Journal of Advanced Nursing*, 14, 833–839.

Kitson, A. (1990) *Quality Patient Care. An Introduction to the Dynamic Standard Setting System*. RCN, Scutari, London.

Moores, B. and Thompson, A.G.H. (1986) What 1357 hospital inpatients think about aspects of their stay in British acute hospitals. *Journal of Advanced Nursing*, 11, 87–102.

Nehring, V. and Geach, B. (1973) Patients' evaluation of their care: why they don't complain. *Nursing Outlook*, 21 (5), 317–321.

Peterson, C. and Stunkard, A.J. (1989) Personal control and health promotion. *Social Science and Medicine*, 28 (8), 814–828.

Rogers, A., Pilgrim, D. and Lacy, R. (1993) *Experiencing Psychiatry. Users' Views of Services*. Macmillan, Basingstoke.

Shields, P.J., Morrison, P. and Hart, D. (1988) Consumer satisfaction on a psychiatric ward. *Journal of Advanced Nursing*, 13, 396–400.

Thompson, D. (1989) Management of the patient with acute myocardial infarction. *Nursing Standard*, 4, 34–38.

Wilkin, D., Hallam, L. and Goggett, M-A. (1992) *Measures of Need and Outcome in Primary Health Care*. Oxford University Press, Oxford.

Chapter 7
Patients' personal concerns assumed great importance

> My clinical work, again centred on the psychological and social aspects of chronic medical illness...I write here to explain to patients, their families, and their practitioners what I have learned from a career passionately devoted to this interest. I write because I wish to popularise a technical literature that would be of great practical value for those who must live with, make sense of, and care for chronic illness. Indeed, I will argue that the study of the experience of illness has something fundamental to teach each of us about the human condition, with its universal suffering and death (Kleinman, 1988).

Introduction

Nurses are constantly reminded of the importance of 'holistic' and 'individualized' care. As a qualified practitioner you will be responsible for drawing up care plans that reflect the needs of individual patients. Holistic care means that carers try to take account of the physical, psychological and social aspects of the patient's life while the patient is hospitalized and dependent to some degree on professional help. Nurses and other healthcare workers try to provide care for the individual patient in these three spheres of living.

In practice, a nurse must take account of a wide range of problems and issues that can affect the patient's health. The complexity and demanding nature of the role often means that nurses give only 'lip service' to some of these facets of a patient's life and the end result is an emphasis on one of these areas of care. In general hospitals it is often the physical aspects of care that are emphasized. However, if nurses really want to provide high-quality care then they must also address the other facets of a patient's life, because a patient's psycho- logical state can affect their physical well-being. For example, if a patient is over-anxious about something at home, he or she will experience more pain. The layout and organization of this major theme is similar to the structure provided in earlier chapters.

PATIENTS' PERSONAL CONCERNS ASSUMED GREAT IMPORTANCE

This was the fourth and final major theme to emerge from the interviews with patients. The 'personal concerns of the patient' both inside and outside the hospital can and often do assume great importance in the patient's life. These personal concerns may not always be recognized by the nurse. In the earlier chapter it was noted that students and qualified nurses gen- erally do not spend a great deal of time with patients. This is also true in the field of mental health nursing, where it might be anticipated that nurses would spend a great deal more of the working day interacting with patients in a therapeutic way (see for example Towell, 1975; Cormack, 1976). It is only by spending time with patients that nurses can learn more about them and therefore provide care tailored to meet those patients' needs.

The personal concern of patients may influence the patients' perceptions of his or her world and their reactions to the immediate context in which care is experienced. In the follow- ing sections some of the issues that emerged during the research interviews with hospitalized patients are explored. These cannot reflect the concerns of *all* patients, but it is nevertheless interesting to note how the patients were willing to share these concerns with me as an unfamiliar researcher visiting the ward environment on an occasional basis. Their concerns had not been discussed with the nurses on the ward. The patients' concerns do give a flavour of the sorts of personal issues and accounts that focus patients' thoughts and feelings and which may be a constant source of often unrecognized anxiety.

(a) The treatment was primary

Many patients perceived their *treatment* as being of the utmost importance and perhaps the most important aspect of being in hospital—having the right treatment was the important thing. Patients may see the nurses' role as simply one of ensuring that patients get the right treatment. This was certainly the case with James, who was only concerned about his treatment—nothing else mattered to him. Ed likewise just needed an operation to put things right, then he could get out of the hospital and resume his normal life outside.

Patients felt that they could not afford to miss out on treatment and several patients saw the role of the hospital (and that included the staff who worked there) as one of 'diagnosis' and 'cure'. When things go wrong with a person's health, the role of the hospital and the staff is simply to put it right. This emphasis on 'cure' reflects perhaps the particular sample of patients who took part in the study, but it may also be a reflection of the views of society in general. The expectations in society of 'what can be done' are becoming greater and greater and this may place a huge burden on staff.

In one way this emphasis on treatment may seem rather egocentric, but the perspective is one that nurses may not fully appreciate. Many nurses are constantly striving to expand their role and incorporate interpersonal and counselling skills, educational initiatives and research-based practice. It may appear that patients do not appreciate efforts to develop the professional standing of nursing. Some, perhaps most, patients are not interested in developments in the nursing profession because they cannot see a link between developments in nursing practice and their 'treatment'. However, if we really do want to 'listen' to the patients' point of view then we must be prepared to accept that many patients will adopt this perspective and respect it. Part of the nurse's task then may be to educate patients and demonstrate how developments in nursing can positively influence their health.

If nurses do recognize this perspective as a valid one, then they can also make an effort to improve the quality of *that individual's care* by being well informed about his or her treatment and medical management and ensure that patients are kept up-to-date. The importance of the nurse's role in giving information to patients and their relatives has been widely demonstrated and discussed earlier (see for example Devine and Cook, 1983). Giving information to patients is also one aspect of nursing that nurses perceive themselves to be good at (Morrison and Burnard, 1991). It is notable, however, that many official complaints about care concern the area of 'information' or rather the lack of information received when in professional care (Audit Commission, 1993).

This general theme should also warn of the dangers of becoming 'too psychological' in the nursing approach to patients. Nurses need to keep a sense of perspective on the nurse–patient relationship and avoid swinging from one extreme (focusing purely on nursing tasks) to the other (focusing on the person and ignoring the tasks that need to be completed safely and competently). The research literature shows that there is a need to improve some facets of psychological care, such as information giving, attitudes and making clinical judgements. However, efforts to do this must be tempered with the knowledge that many patients see the *treatment as primary*. They just want to get better and go home to their families.

Patients need to be confident that nurses and doctors know what they are 'doing' and are competent to perform 'skilled tasks and procedures'. All this suggests to me that in training nurses and other healthcare workers we ought to be looking at ways to *link* the 'basic and more technical' skills that a competent practitioner must have with the psychological approach and skills that will also enhance his or her performance and make the patient feel like a 'person worthy of care'. Nurse educators and practitioners need to develop educational packages that integrate these skills and attitudes.

(b) Being in hospital was frustrating

Being in hospital can be a very frustrating time for patients. The patient's whole life has been altered by illness. Their work, social life and personal relationships have been seriously disrupted. In some cases, such as life-threatening illness, unexpected trauma or the diagnosis of a stigmatizing illness such as breast cancer or schizophrenia, a person's life may be ruined. Nurses experience a wide range of professional work environments and learn how to feel comfortable being there. Many nurses are happy to work in traumatic and stressful work situations. Patients are different. They are in hospital because they have to be there; they have very little choice. While some patients may be in hospital for investigations and are obviously not acutely 'ill', others may be there for life-saving surgery, to have children, or for more long-term treatment.

Hospitals are places where rules and regulations dominate. These are necessary to ensure that the institution functions effectively. Some rules are explicit—do not smoke. Other rules are tacitly implied—all patients must wear night attire in a general surgical ward. Sometimes informal rules, such as the wearing of night clothes, dressing gown and slippers, are applied generally and these may heighten the frustration that a patient feels. Short-stay patients or patients who are not acutely ill may be required to stay in bed or in night clothes. This can be disheartening, particularly if they have to observe other people who are acutely ill, in severe pain or dying.

Frustration can result from different sources. That a person's life is temporarily disrupted may be bad enough, but having to ask a nurse for a 'bottle' may be both embarrassing and frustrating. One of the patients, Hugh, was disheartened because he felt quite well in himself but he *had to stay in bed*. Using a commode beside the bed in a ward with other patients may be particularly anxiety-provoking. Many patients in hospital may be able to look after themselves. They are often referred to as 'self-caring' during the daily report because they do not need much direct nursing. Yet these individuals are often subject to the same restrictive regimes that many acutely ill patients willingly undergo without question.

Other patients may be frustrated at being in hospital for lengthy periods, especially when nothing appears to be happening. The days and nights were boring for some patients. Nurses must learn to think about the needs of each individual patient and be prepared to organize a more 'flexible' regime of care according to the needs and abilities of these individual patients. Boredom and inactivity are major sources of patient frustration and irritation that can often be dealt with successfully with a little careful planning and imagination.

(c) Felt let down by the GP after husband's death
During her interview Florence talked a lot about her general practitioner (GP) who was very supportive when her husband died. She felt that he was one of those doctors who was 'always available and willing to talk' to her about the death of her husband and her own health. Since her husband died, Florence too had become ill and needed to make more frequent calls on the GP service. As time went by, Florence began to feel 'neglected' and 'let down' by the GP practice; she felt let down by her own doctor especially and also by the other doctors in the practice, most of whom lacked patience with her.

In the end, Florence had to become more assertive. She 'insisted' that her doctor made an appointment with the consultant surgeon at the local hospital because she was convinced that something was seriously wrong even though the doctors at the GP practice were not. They seemed to think that her health difficulties were more 'psychological' and a reaction to the death of her husband. Eventually Florence did see the consultant surgeon and this led to her admission to hospital for surgery.

This scenario is perhaps not that uncommon. Patients need to be able to talk things through and re-establish themselves as individuals worthy of the care that health workers provide. All too often these sorts of concerns that 'worry' patients are never mentioned and resolved successfully. The sorts of experiences that Florence had with her GP practice can also seriously undermine a person's confidence in other forms of health services. If patients have little trust and confidence in the professional carers who are paid to look after them, how can we expect patients to comply with health education advice and treatment regimes that promote health?

(d) Mother's recent death

Eileen recounted how her mother had died recently, just before she had to come into hospital. Eileen had to deal with the death, the funeral and its aftermath, and this experience continued to play a very significant part in Eileen's life even though she now found herself in hospital and in need of treatment. On admission she was 'very ill'. Now that she was feeling better she had time to think. Her mother's death made her think carefully about her own care in hospital and the care given to other elderly patients like her mother. She found herself 'observing the ward' and the staff to see what they did for the patients. It changed her views about the way hospitals cared for the elderly in the community. She was not sure any more if hospital was the best place for old people who were dying.

This is a particularly good example of the nurses' need to take account of the important things that may be happening or have recently happened to a person who arrives on the ward as a patient. People who are bereaved usually need to talk to others about it. The bereavement enters every aspect of a person's life and may be thought about constantly. Nurses may need to set aside time to talk to the patient, and this background material will help the nurses to meet a particular patient's needs and draw up an appropriate plan of care. However, this is a difficult thing to do and anxiety-provoking, and it may cause some conflict between colleagues with a more 'detached' approach to patients (Menzies, 1970).

(e) The previous admission to hospital was terrible

As a nurse we may see the patient as a new admission to our ward or unit. We can forget that many patients may have a 'patient career', which can span several years and numerous admissions. Previous admissions and experiences of hospital life can affect the patients' perceptions of what to expect and how he or she will be treated. They can help the patient to come into hospital in a more stable state of mind or they can generate crippling anxiety.

One patient, George, described his previous admission to hospital for major surgery for a damaged kidney. It was a very disappointing experience. George was recovering from the surgery, but was discharged before he had made a full recovery because the hospital needed to free up beds for patients awaiting admission. The staff were very concerned about the shortage of beds. At the time he was discharged, George did not feel well enough to go home but *his* views were not asked for. The doctor discharged him anyway. Worse was to come— the results of the investigations performed in hospital were not sent to George's GP, which made the management of his condition all the more arbitrary and uncertain at home. That last admission was a 'terrible' experience for George.

Such previous experiences may weaken the confidence that patients and their families have in professional caring services. They highlight the need for nurses to ensure that they know each individual patient by becoming familiar with their medical notes and asking those patients about their earlier experiences of hospital and the treatment they received from professional staff. Such an approach will help to promote a more sensitive and effective management of each individual patient. It will help staff to ensure that care is personalized and holistic.

(f) Concerned about the family and close friends
The final topic to emerge as an important aspect of the patients' personal concerns dealt with their families and friends. At times of illness, people get physical and psychological support from other family members. These family members, friends or partners may provide different forms of social support for patients. For many patients these supporting mechanisms work very well. Unfortunately other patients do not have this type of support and they may themselves be the major supportive force in the lives of others outside of the hospital.

Professional helpers naturally enough often see the patient as *the* member of the family who is in crisis. Some patients, however, may be especially concerned about the health and well-being of the other family members who are *not* in hospital. Martha's mother, for example, lived over 250 miles away from the hospital and she herself needed an operation to save the sight in her one good eye. She needed Martha to care for her, but Martha was stranded in hospital with no chance of a quick discharge. Martha's mother and her husband were all the family she had, and being far away from them was a 'constant source of worry'.

Another elderly patient, Ed, was very concerned for the one 'visitor' who came to see him everyday. She had to travel into the hospital by public transport and this meant she had to have two changes of bus. It took over an hour to get to the hospital. It was a long way for an elderly person and the travelling took up much of her day. Ed was grateful that she came to see him, but he was 'worried about her health' because she had arthritis in her leg and was 'not very good on her feet'. She found it very difficult to get around and waiting for buses in bad weather was not good for her. Ed 'worried' about her.

In the busy hospital environment these personal concerns for others outside hospital may often go unrecognized by nurses and doctors. Not every patient had to deal with these 'personal concerns', but for those who did, they were very real sources of anxiety and uncertainty.

The few issues mentioned here may appear to some as rather minor, but think for a moment about some of the patient concerns you may have come across: dependent or disabled relatives living at home, the effect of long-term illness on future employment opportunities, patients with small children to look after at home, financial crisis, animals left unattended, worries about a spouse's ability to cope with running a home alone, and so on. These are just some of the issues that can be sources of additional anxiety in hospitalized patients. These types of issues may influence the ways that patients react to illness and treatment.

Personal concerns of the patient

This was the last major theme to emerge from the interviews with patients. It provided more details about the patients' lifeworld. It highlighted other details about the patients' experiences that were very personal to the patient. These issues may assume great importance for the patient in hospital, but may be of little interest to, or not noticed by, the staff. The personal concerns of the patients, however, served as important reminders of life outside the hospital and the need for patients to continue to deal with current issues and relationships outside.

The patients' personal concerns emphasized the sorts of difficulties that relatives or friends of the patients often have to deal with. The issues described here focus the patients' attention on the outside world. The treatment was a primary concern. They wanted to get better and get out of this place— nothing more, nothing less. These patients saw their stay in hospital as an ordeal that had to be tolerated. Relationships with staff were of little importance except that some contact with staff was essential to ensure that the treatment programmes were adhered to. Getting better was the most important thing in their lives.

One patient, Hugh, was frustrated at being in hospital because he did not feel particularly ill. Nobody wanted to be in hospital unnecessarily. His frustration was heightened by the fact that he felt as though he was treated like an object in hospital (see Chapter 4). Florence was very upset by the behaviour of her GP and his colleagues in the practice. The recent death of Eileen's mother was upsetting and in hospital she had time to think about it and her own future. She was unsure about what would become of her now. George thought about his previous admission to hospital, which was terrible. He contrasted that admission with his present experience of hospital, which was much better. Other patients were worried about their family and close friends; they felt cut off and lonely.

Emotionally upset during the interviews

During the interviews some of the patients became very emotional and tearful when they talked about their personal concerns: the distances their relatives had to travel just to visit them, or the problems of relatives' ill health, and how responsible and guilty they felt while in hospital. Other patients did not become overtly tearful, but they were upset. It was obvious that these concerns were important for the patients and must have influenced the way they responded to and reacted to hospital.

Four of the 10 patients became emotionally upset during the interviews and cried for a very short period. All quickly regained their composure and continued with the interview; they did not want to stop the interview. After the tape recorder was switched off I sat with these patients for a short while and talked with them generally. On leaving the ward I mentioned to the nurse in charge that the patient had become upset and asked if someone could check on the patient later on. It is still unclear why these patients became emotionally upset during the interviews because the focus of the interviews was not an especially difficult or sensitive area. One possible explanation may be that another person, even a stranger doing research, actually *took time to talk to them* about their illness, their experiences and themselves. This intervention alone may have emphasized the intensely vulnerable position in which these individuals found themselves.

In an earlier chapter it was noted that none of these patients developed close relationships with nurses. They had few opportunities to express their anxieties to the staff and to deal with this successfully. In the research, the patients were given a chance to tell someone about their experiences in hospital. The time and interest showed during the interviews seemed to be the stimulus for eliciting the rich and detailed responses that must form the basis of any attempt to provide individualized nursing care for patients.

What can be done to improve the situation

Practitioners can do several things to help patients here. The need to *make time to talk* to patients is very significant. However, it is also important to guard against a tendency to 'interrogate' the patient in one short burst during the admission procedure. To do so is likely to *heighten anxiety* at a time when patients are already very anxious. It may be better if nurses plan the time that they need to spend with patients so that thay 'visit' the patient on different occasions throughout the duration of the admission, collecting relevant information in an incremental fashion. This planned strategy will allow the relationship to develop at a *natural pace* so that relevant information may be collected as the nurse builds up a good rapport with each new patient. This may be very hard to do, especially if the ward is a short-stay ward. Nevertheless, it is a strategy that will prove to be more successful in helping nurses to collect the information needed to plan patient care.

Another strategy is to invite friends or relatives of the patient to talk about the patient's home circumstances and any worries they have about the home situation. They can often provide vital clues about a patient's suitability for discharge and the likelihood of success at home after hospitalization. If any information about the patient casts a doubt about the success of his or her recovery following discharge, then links with other professionals, such as social workers, occupational therapists or physiotherapists, can help to explore potential problems more fully. Collaboration of this nature between different healthcare workers will promote effective care both in hospital and in the patient's home.

It should be clear, even from these few interviews, that patients' lives are complex. Nurses often have to deal with the lives of many different patients at the same time. It is not feasible or realistic to expect to be able to handle all the professional and personal information that a ward of 30 patients may generate. Learn to work with colleagues to structure the work and reorganize it into teams or groups. Many well-organized wards use this approach already to good effect.

Summary

In this short chapter some of the personal issues that can and do affect the psychological well-being of patients in care have been described. If nurses and other healthcare workers wish to practise holistic and individualized care, then they must be prepared to set aside time for patients and listen carefully to what they say. Not all patients will want to do this. Some will be more concerned with receiving the correct treatment and leaving hospital as quickly as possible. This is probably a healthy sign.

Nevertheless some patients will need a little extra care and attention to help them through a very difficult stage of their lives. Only a few of the concerns of patients have been mentioned here. It is likely that as you focus on this sort of approach to patient care, you will uncover many more. By acknowledging the existence of these concerns in the patient's life you have already prepared yourself to work towards helping patients to deal effectively with these potential problem areas.

Further reading

Abel, E. (1987) *Love is not Enough. Family Care of the Frail Elderly*. American Public Health Association, Washington.

Archbold, P.G. (1983) Impact of parent-caring on women. *Family Relations*, 32, 39–45.

Braithwaite, V.A. (1990) *Bound to Care*. Allen and Unwin, London.

Cartwright, A., Hockey, L. and Anderson, J.L. (1973) *Life Before Death*. Routledge, London.

Engelhardt, H.T. Jr (1982) Illnesses, diseases, and sicknesses. In: V. Kestenbaum (ed.) *The Humanity of the Ill: Phenomenological Perspectives*. University of Tennessee Press, Knoxville, pp. 142–156.

Kestenbaum, V. (ed.) (1982) *The Humanity of the Ill: Phenomenological Perspectives*. University of Tennessee Press, Knoxville.

Kobasa, S.C.O., Maddi, S.R., Pucetti, M.C. and Zola, M.A. (1985) Effectiveness of hardiness, exercise and social support as resources against illness. *Journal of Psychosomatic Research*, 29, 525–533.

Luria, A.R. (1975) *The Man With a Shattered World. A History of a Brain Wound*. (Translated from the Russian by Lynn Solotaroff.) Penguin, Harmondsworth.

Pulling, J. (1987) *The Caring Trap*. Fontana, London.

Sacks, O. (1985) *The Man Who Mistook His Wife For a Hat*. Picador, London.

Toombs, S.K. (1992) *The Meaning of Illness. A Phenomenological Account of the Different Perspectives of Physician and Patient*. Kluwer, London.

Chapter 8
Critical issues in the caring relationship

> ... the concept of caring stands as a critique of the way in which nursing, remedial therapies and social work have developed not only to provide tending services but also as part of the regulatory institutions of society, in which the interests of the state are those of dominant classes. So the caring professions can be seen to exercise power not only through skilled practices which meet the needs of their clientele but also through state sponsorship (with its attendant constraints) that provides the institutional basis for those practices (Hugman, 1991).

Introduction

The relationship between patients and nurses is complex. The patient enters into the relationship because he or she is ill and needs help. The nurse and other healthcare workers are there to help in a skilled and professional way. In the last four chapters some of the important themes that form the patients' experiences of being cared for have been examined. This chapter discusses some of the wider issues that emerged as the patients' experiences were described. These issues influence the nurse–patient relationship, and other professional–patient relationships, at the practice level.

Power

The issue of 'power' in the nurse–patient relationship is important because it may cast a shadow over what nurses do. Morse (1991) reported a research study in which interviews with 86 nurses were analysed using the grounded theory approach. A major theme to emerge from the analysis was the idea of 'negotiating the relationship' between the patient and the nurse. The negotiation process was found to generate 'involvement' and 'commitment'. However, Morse did not mention the fact that any form of negotiation must occur from different perspectives. If the perspectives were the same there would be no need to negotiate.

In the scenario described in this book, the patient is in a *very vulnerable* position while the nurse is in a position of *control and power*. These different positions were clearly highlighted in the study outlined here, but they have also been recognized in other studies involving patients (see for example Robinson, 1968; May, 1990). The impact of the status and social position of the individuals participating in these negotiations must be more fully understood if we are to develop helpful relationships with patients. This is particularly important in those areas of nursing where a physical illness is not the major reason why the nurse and the patient come together. In many areas of mental health nursing, for example, there is less pressure on time and it is expected that the nurse will base his or her care on the 'relationship' with the patient.

In another chapter it was noted that one of the patients always addressed the nurses as 'nurse' no matter how well he knew the nurse involved. This had the effect of reinforcing the unequal status that separated the nurse and the patient. It was an overt mechanism for displaying deference to the staff. This type of relationship is obviously not one of equals because the professional carer seems to be 'giving' all the time and receiving little in return. This is not strictly true. The deferential mode of presentation adopted by many patients may well serve as a means of legitimizing the professional and caring role of the nurse and other professional carers (Kelly and May,

1982; May and Kelly, 1982). The legitimization process may be enough to make the relationship between the nurse and patient more 'reciprocal' (Rempusheski *et al.*, 1988). The need to 'pay back' the carers has been described elsewhere as an attitude of 'indebtedness' (Greenberg and Westcott, 1982).

Social exchange theory is another psychological theory that can help us to understand some aspects of the nurse–patient relationship (Baron and Byrne, 1987). The theory states that social behaviour (helping other people) may be considered in terms of *rewards* and *costs* that are governed by the norms of *equity*. These norms emerge in society so that when an individual helps another individual, he or she can expect to be rewarded according to the cost of the effort needed to help that other person. Note that the professional context in which people get paid to 'care' may change the way in which the theory can be understood.

The rewards–costs equation needs to be kept in a state of *balance*; if it is not, then the helper may experience distress— anxiety, stress, burnout. When a balance is achieved and people feel they have been treated fairly, they are more likely to be cooperative. In normal social interaction some individuals may try to minimize their costs and maximize their benefits. In the nursing context, the costs of establishing and maintaining caring relationships with patients is constantly reviewed by hospital staff (Morrison, 1991, 1992). Although the work of the nurse is recognized as being very 'stressful', many nurses receive a very powerful sense of job and personal satisfaction through helping others in hospital. The costs and rewards equation is therefore kept in a state of balance. The nurse, because of her position within an institutional hierarchy, remains in a powerful position.

It is also interesting to note how the staff in this study used the first names of the patients when interacting with patients. Many staff took the liberty of calling patients by their first names even though many of the patients were older and more senior than the nurses. Permission to do so was rarely sought, and even if it was, patients were unlikely to say 'no' because this would identify them as 'different' from other members of the patient group. This strategy too may empower the staff and increase their status over the patients. However, it must be acknowledged that some patients liked being called by their first names because it made them feel 'human', even if it meant being an extremely vulnerable and dependent human. The nurses were also empowered to touch patients and perform intimate and highly personal tasks. This ability was never questioned by patients.

The demeanour of both patients and staff (Goffman, 1956) also played a role in determining the behaviour of nurses and patients. The patients were always dressed in night attire, although only one or two of them really needed to be at the time of the interviews. The nurses were dressed in their uniforms, which immediately displayed their grade and level of expertise to patients and visitors to the ward. The demeanour of the patients and nurses helped to reinforce the differences in status and position in the hospital set-up.

Power in the professional helping relationship

Not surprisingly the issue of power in professional helping relationships has not been researched in any depth. It goes against the very things that nurses and other professional helpers, such as clinical psychologists, counsellors, social workers and doctors, aspire to in practice: focusing on 'people' rather than 'patients', encouraging people to assume responsibility for their health, getting people to be involved in decisions about their treatment and so on. However, a small number of writers have however, noted the possible influence of power in the helper–client relationship.

Guggenbühl-Craig (1971) described an analysis of the work of professional carers and helpers including therapists, doctors and social workers that revealed a *desire for power over clients* amongst these professional groups. Criticisms of the established and accepted ways of receiving care have been hard-hitting. Some even go so far as to suggest that patients are 'exploited'. In a discussion of the consequences of institutionalized care for the sick person, Parsons (1951) noted that:

> ... the combination of helplessness, lack of technical competence, and emotional disturbance make him a peculiarly vulnerable object for exploitation (p. 445).

In a direct attack on the professional medical healthcare system Illich (1975) stated that:

> A professional and physician-based health care system which has grown beyond tolerable bounds is sickening for these reasons: it must produce clinical damages which outweigh its potential benefits; it cannot but obscure the political conditions which rendered society unhealthy; and it tends to expropriate the power of the individual to heal himself and to shape his or her environment (p. 11).

Illich also describes three types of 'iatrogenesis' that resulted from an inappropriate amount of power in the hands of doctors. Iatrogenesis refers to illness that has been *caused* by the staff, the treatment or the hospital environment. The severe side-effects of drugs used to treat people are one form of iatrogenic illness. The different forms of iatrogenic illness described by Illich include: social iatrogenesis (the promotion of dependence on care, drugs and other forms of medical technology); and structural iatrogenesis (characterized by the individual's loss of power over his or her own life and health).

Clearly, nurses also hold power over patients and the desire for 'nursing' to become more 'professional' can only increase this power. Great care is needed if we are to develop in ways that enhance patient care. Nurses must not forget that their primary role is to look after patients. Professional developments in education and research are important, but they must be guided by the need to improve direct care in different areas.

The ideal of mutuality

Mutuality is closely related to the power issue. Companionship suggests mutuality. In accompanying another person we share the relationship and each supports and helps the other. The *degree* to which this is possible in the nursing field is a matter of some contention. Carl Rogers (1967) suggested that the relationship between the individual being helped and the helper *is a mutual one* in therapy.

This is surely an ideal to aim at that cannot be fully realized in a professional helping context. The philosopher Martin Buber (1966) suggested that because the patient comes to the professional for help, the relationship can *never be a mutual one*. On the question of mutuality he wrote:

> He comes for help to you. You don't come for help to him.
> And not only this, but you are *able*, more or less, to help him.
> He can do different things to you, but not help you ... You
> are, of course, a very important person for him. But not a
> person whom he wants to see and to know and is able to ...
> He is, may I say, entangled in your life, in your thoughts, in
> your being, your communication, and so on. But he is not
> interested in you as you. It cannot be. You are interested in ...
> in him as this person. This kind of detached presence he
> cannot have and give (Buber, 1966, p. 171).

The issue of mutuality has been discussed in detail elsewhere (Friedman, 1985), yet it is one that will continue to be debated. It is difficult to see how 'mutuality' could be achieved in practice except in cases where a long-term relationship between the patient and the nurse has developed and has been maintained over time. Many of the issues discussed in Chapter

3—learned helplessness, attributions, the sick role and illness behaviour as well as the organizational structure and culture— will underpin the nurse–patient relationship.

In an earlier chapter patients were described as being extremely anxious about being 'treated like an object' while in hospital. Some of the patients were ignored as people and their personal details were discussed publicly. In contrast, other patients commented on the positive effect of being 'treated like a person' while in hospital. It helped to promote recovery and made them feel good in themselves. This distinction made by several patients is similar to the I–It and I–Thou types of relationships described by Martin Buber (1958) and is also an essential part of the concept of mutuality. Several authors have discussed some of the issues surrounding this process at length (Goffman, 1968; Van den Berg, 1972b; Gadow, 1980; Drew, 1986).

This theme of crushing vulnerability was vividly highlighted by two patients involved in the research who developed cancer and which assumed great importance in their lives. Finding out about the cancer had a shattering impact on both patients. They had to face their fears about death and dying and learn somehow to cope with the diagnosis and whatever the future had in store for them.

Other patients faced traumatic investigations or surgery or had their operations cancelled at the last minute. One patient harboured an anxious suspicion about his condition. Another patient became very distressed by the fact that she had to surrender her independence to the staff. Some patients were lonely and felt forgotten about, while another felt like a smelly mess compared with the young nurses who looked after her. All these aspects of the patients' lifeworld heightened other feelings of being made to feel like an object and the positive effects of being treated like a person worthy of care and attention.

Commitment

The relationship between informal or unpaid carers and those they care for has been examined from other perspectives. A crucial element of the relationship between the informal carer and the cared for person is *commitment*. Kitson (1987b) argued that commitment is a vital component of the professional caring relationship found in nursing. This was also identified in another part of the study described here, as part of what I called 'the caring attitude' (Morrison, 1991). In that part of the study, caring nurses were perceived as having a wide range of 'attitudinal characteristics', including 'commitment' in the form of a specific category called 'level of motivation'. The categories were as follows:

- personal qualities (kindness, genuineness)
- clinical work style (treats people as individuals, explains treatment and care to patients)
- interpersonal approach (sensitive approach, listens to people)
- level of motivation (highly motivated, conscientious)
- concern for others (puts others before self, concerned for people)
- use of time (always has time for people, has time for supporting relationships)
- attitudes (consistent in attitude, down to earth attitude).

The level of commitment has also been found to be a crucial determinant in research studies of informal carers (Goodman, 1986). Although caring for disabled relatives in the community has been found to exact a heavy toll on carers, it was suggested that commitment was a prerequisite for *mutuality* in the caring situation. In a study of family caregiving, Hirschfeld (1983) claimed that:

... mutuality between the supportive and the impaired family
members emerged as the major parameter for families
managing life with senile brain disease. In the face of
immense problems posed by the impact of the decline itself,
the implications of caring for a senile brain diseased person
and the difficulties rooted in the social environment, mutuality
became *the* important variable (p. 26).

Despite being under tremendous pressures and strain, successful care-givers gained a great deal from their relationships with
the impaired persons. The level of commitment that they
displayed gave their lives meaning, purpose and understanding. It should be noted that in these studies the informal carers
were not 'paid' to care. The commitment involved and the
nature of the relationship between the carer and the patient is
(in my view) quite different from the professional context. It is
unrealistic to expect the same level of 'personal commitment'
from professional helpers compared with the personal commitment entailed in caring for a dependent husband or wife when
the couple have been married for a long time. The nature of the
relationship is quite different.

It has been argued that the role of the nurse is to assume
responsibility for the care of a person when the lay or informal
carer can no longer cope (Kitson, 1987a, b). The ability of the
nurse to integrate the attributes of lay-caring into the pro-
fessional-caring relationship will facilitate the development of
a mutually experienced relationship. This can have a direct
bearing on the quality of care received as follows:

Quality of care in the professional caring relationship is
thought to relate to the extent to which aspects of caring
activities implicit in the lay-caring relationship are carried into
the professional nurse/patient relationship and made explicit.
The ability of the nurse to do this emerges as one aspect of the
therapeutic function (Kitson, 1987b, p. 155).

However, it is not at all certain if a 'mutual' relationship can be achieved in a professional context. The small scale findings presented in this book cast serious doubt on the possibility of a 'mutual' nurse–patient relationship. The descriptions of the patients' experiences may be interpreted in line with the theoretical descriptions outlined in Chapter 3. To expect professional carers to display the same level of commitment as a long-term informal carer is to place a great burden on staff and generate feelings of failure. However, there is a great need for further research into this area before any firm conclusions can be drawn.

A number of important questions must be addressed before policy and practice are challenged and changed. The following list of questions ought to be considered first: Can the level of commitment required of a paid nurse ever be the same as a relative? Does it need to be? How does the nurse benefit from the relationship? Can the nurse always be a professional carer? What personal processes influence the professional context? How supportive is the professional team for the individual nurse? It is only by researching these sorts of questions that we come to understand the nature of the nurse–patient relationship more fully. Through that understanding we will be able to care more effectively for those people in our care.

The importance of physical care

The importance of the physical care of the patient must not be overlooked as the profession develops. The importance of 'physical' or 'basic' nursing care in caring for the person as a 'whole' emerged following interviews with nurses and patients. There is an obvious yet *crucial link* between physical and psychological nursing care because the need to complete basic care tasks means that a nurse *must spend time with a patient*. This time presents the nurse with an opportunity to interact with the patient while completing some basic care tasks. However, in practice, the basic care is often carried out by untrained nurses and students. In effect, the least well-trained staff are the ones who have most contact with patients.

It seems strange that the most experienced and highly qualified members of the nursing workforce, those best equipped to provide psychological care, have such limited contact with patients. Hence their psychological care of patients is not linked up with the provision of basic nursing care. They are missing important opportunities for providing psychological care. In another research study of medical and surgical nurses in a German hospital, a similar picture emerged (Morrison and Bauer, 1993), while Smith (1992) stated that:

> The patient makes clear links between the emotional and physical aspects of her care. She describes caring gestures, the little things that make her feel qualitatively different: nurses who recognised she needed to talk, were good listeners, held her hand, took away her fear and had a calming influence on her. She described them as 'brilliant' indicating that she recognised they had skills, but also implied that these caring gestures were 'natural' ... Emotional labour does make a difference and care matters to patients, but it is still in danger of being marginalised (p. 145).

Patients also need technically competent nurses and doctors to look after them. There is a need for balance between the necessity for good technical, basic care and psychological care (Benner, 1984). These three areas should be closely linked in training because they are the requirements of a good nurse.

When nurses give direct physical or basic care (and technical care to a lesser extent), they are provided with a *bridge* for giving psychological care to the patient. Trained practising nurses themselves recognize this, but continue to emphasize the 'managerial' aspects of the role, which assume greater importance within the organizational hierarchy and culture (Morrison, 1991, 1992). Trained nurses need to refocus on the link between the physical and psychological care of the patient to provide individualized care for the whole patient. There is also a need for educators to develop ways of teaching students how to provide psychological care at the same time as providing basic care for patients. One possible approach that might be helpful here is to incorporate the 'problem-based learning' strategy into educational courses.

The principal idea behind problem-based learning is '... that the starting point for learning should be a problem, a query or puzzle that the learner wishes to solve' (Boud, 1985, p. 13). This approach has enormous potential, and not just for nursing and psychology teaching. If the problem-based approach is implemented effectively it can help the student to build a 'bridge' between a range of *theoretical* disciplines such as psychology, sociology, pharmacology and anatomy and the *practical* problems that comprise the work of the practising nurse.

There is also a need for managers of nursing services to address the issue of the psychological care of patients. The stated aim of most nursing units is to provide 'quality care', and that includes physical and psychological aspects of care. Clearly, time is needed to build good relationships. If more trained nurses are to become involved in direct patient care, then managers must take account of that fact and begin to change the culture of organizations so that basic care is not seen as low-status work to be left to the untrained staff. Changing organizations will also have financial implications, but changes in work practice can be achieved by helping individual practitioners to work in a different way. These changes will need the support of the managers within the organizations.

What has emerged from this study most powerfully is the significance of caring for the whole person. Individual nurses, and particularly trained nurses, must try to reimmerse themselves in direct caring activities. The trained nurses of today were students yesterday. However, as trained and more experienced nurses they have assumed higher status and power and many have alienated themselves from the patient. This orientation may or may not be different in other branches of nursing and health care, and therefore these other branches also need to be scrutinized carefully. In terms of general adult care, however, the trend described here is widespread (see for example Evers, 1986).

To a large extent this alienation has been brought about by the system of delivering nursing care, with its hierarchical structures and the role of medicine as a model for providing nursing care. Dunlop (1986) noted how the history of the meaning of caring has a:

> ... complex past ... including its negative and lower order associations, which may prove hard to shift, because they are so embedded in the background meanings. It seems to be no accident, in other words, that 'cure' is associated with a high-status, predominantly male occupation, which jealously guards access to the term, while 'care' is relegated to women ... (p. 662).

The separation of nursing care into 'instrumental' (behaviours and tasks) and 'expressive' (attitudes and emotional issues) components may lead to more difficulties by dissecting nursing work into low status (attending to the basic needs of the patient) and high status (administering medicines, doing doctors' ward rounds, administration and so on) tasks. A synthesized perspective has been advocated as follows:

> In caring for sick people, many aspects of whose being-in-the-world become problematic rather than taken for granted, there is a temptation to concentrate either on the troubled body or the troubled psyche in order to simplify nursing work, yet what the nursing community agrees is good nursing is neither purely physical nor purely psychosocial. The nurse must thus find her way between the twin temptations of physicality and disembodiment (Dunlop, 1986, p. 664).

This objective could be realized on an *individual basis* and some nurses seem to have achieved this already. To attempt to refocus institutional care systems is quite another matter. Much time, energy and resources have already been invested in producing the present system of values and customary modes of nursing practice. However, if there is a genuine concern for the consumers of health care then the managers of the system must begin to address the needs of consumers. The rhetoric must match the reality in practice.

Ordinary patients and ordinary nurses

There is a great emphasis in the current literature on psychological care of the patient. Nurses can learn a great deal from the psychological literature and put this into nursing practice. There is no need for all nurses to become 'expert counsellors' in order to help patients. However, there are certainly some essential counselling skills that a nurse must have, e.g. the ability to *listen* to people and to try to *avoid being judgmental*. To become a skilled counsellor would involve additional training and experience. There is, however, a need for some nurses to do this, but to expect all nurses to reach this level of skill is unrealistic. Not every nurse is suited to the counsellor role.

Acquiring some of the important skills and attitudes mentioned in this book will certainly help nurses to be more aware of the psychological care of the patient. The positive effects of being an *ordinary person* who happens to be a nurse helping other ordinary people should not be underestimated. Patients need to know that those looking after them are human too. In a study of informal helping, Cowen (1982) described how members of the public sought help from different occupational groups. The study examined peoples' willingness to discuss 'psychological problems', such as difficulties with children, job insecurity, loneliness, problems with colleagues and depression, with hairdressers, lawyers, supervisors and bartenders rather than seeking out an expert in mental health.

The informal helpers offered a wide range of helpful interventions—they offered support and sympathy, they tried to make light of the problems, they listened, they offered alternative solutions, they shared their personal experiences, they gave advice, they asked questions, they pointed out the consequences of bad ideas or tried to get the person to talk to someone else. All the groups generally felt good about offering this very 'ordinary' service to customers and they believed themselves to be moderately good at it. Nurses should try to develop this 'ordinary' and 'spontaneous' approach in nursing practice.

Dilemmas facing all professional carers

The professional helping relationship, whether it be in nursing, medicine, social work or clinical psychology, is to some extent always going to be undermined by several 'essential conflicts' common to all professional helping relationships. Nursing, as well as other helping professions, must tackle these issues directly if real progress is to be made and the care given is to match up to the stated standards. The most notable of these conflicts have been discussed in depth elsewhere (Lenrow, 1978), so only a brief summary is provided here. Lenrow (1978) included the following issues that lead to conflict:

- There is an inherent contradiction in the term 'professional helper'. People have a natural sympathetic attitude towards others in distress and are willing to help them. To be paid to do this changes the whole nature of the relationship. To be paid to care introduces elements of professional skill and detached involvement (Campbell, 1985). It places limits and boundaries on the helping process.

- Professional helpers are often seen as distant and different from those they claim to help. They are seen as well educated and in control of their lives. The patients they help are often the most vulnerable members of our society: the poor, the unemployed, the elderly, the physically and mentally handicapped, and those with chronic illnesses.

- The values of the professional helping groups are often in conflict with those they claim to help. Professional carers tend to be drawn from middle-class families. The values they hold about education, family life, health, money, politics and so on will be very different from the people they help as part of their professional role (Pendleton and Bochner, 1980).

- The system of 'organized' care also has a direct impact on the individual carer. It is clear that organizational structures and the organizational culture can influence how an individual nurse (or patient) behaves in hospital or as part of a system of caring.

Lenrow goes on to suggest that:

> When a professional's work is embedded in bureaucratic structure, his role may be incompatible with helping, in the sense that many of his actions are not intended to help and that the clients (or students) do not perceive the professional's work as intended to help them (Lenrow, 1978, p. 279).

Further contradictions in the professional helping role arise because the professional carer emphasizes 'technological supremacy' in dealing with the problems that an individual faces. Moreover there is tendency amongst professional helpers to 'blame the victims' for their own misfortunes and ill health—poor housing, inappropriate health education, unemployment, family history of disease, poor diet, lack of exercise, excessive alcohol consumption or cigarette smoking. The attributions made by professional staff may underpin this tendency to apportion blame to patients (see Chapter 3). These and other similar conflicts tend to get in the way of the helping process and affect the way the carer perceives the person he or she is supposed to help.

What can be done to improve the situation

The issues discussed in this chapter influence the nurse–patient relationship. It is widely recognized that there is room for improvement in the provision of psychological care. To do this successfully nurses will need to be more aware of the social world of the institutional setting in which patients are cared for. On a personal level you can ask several key questions to heighten your own awareness of the ward setting. Think about your own status and position in the organizational hierarchy. Observe colleagues at work. Learn to notice where you fit into the ward hierarchy. Who has the *power* to change things? Who do you model yourself on? Who provides the role model for colleagues? Is the unit a very hierarchical one or are people outspoken. Is assertiveness tolerated? How do patients respond to being on the ward? Are they 'good' or 'bad' patients? Is there a happy atmosphere on the ward that both patients and staff appreciate? Can junior members of staff challenge established norms? Or do people do things unquestioningly? Are staff highly motivated?

As a nurse, think about how you give care. If you are involved in giving direct care to patients, ask yourself if you make the most of the opportunities you have for giving good psychological care at the same time. As you give a patient a bed bath do you *talk* to the patient? Do you *listen* to the patient? Do you familiarize yourself with the patient's condition and progress *before* you approach the patient so that you are up-to-date with all the relevant information about him or her? Have you learned to relax with patients? To be ordinary in the way you interact? Have you learned how to give information effectively so that it will not be forgotten or misunderstood? Do you remember to check for understanding when you give patients important information? Do you try to involve patients in planning care? Do you encourage patients to take responsibility and make decisions? These are just some of the things you ought to think about to implement improvements in your nursing care.

Summary

In this chapter some of the more abstract ideas that can directly influence the care that patients receive in hospital have been explored. The power that the professional carer holds over patients is obvious and runs counter to the aspirations of many professional carers: promoting independence and giving personal responsibility for health back to the patients themselves.

The notion of mutuality is, as we have seen, an important facet of many long-term informal caring relationships, which gives meaning to the lives of the carers. The level of commitment found in professional caring relationships cannot be equated with that often found with informal carers. The costs and the rewards involved in informal and formal helping relationships are quite different. There are, however, many parallels between the informal and formal (professional) caring roles. The 'skilled companionship' that Campbell referred to seems to be a sensible compromise and more realistic basis for nursing patients.

Further reading

Botelho, R.J. (1992) A negotiation model for the doctor–patient relationship. *Family Practice*, 9 (2), 210–218.
Boud, D. (1985) Problem-based learning in perspective. In: D.

Boud (ed.) *Problem Based Learning in Education for the Professions*. Higher Education Research and Development Society of Australasia, Sydney, pp. 13–18.

Campbell, A.V. (1984) *Moderated Love. A Theology of Professional Care*. SPCK, London.

Campbell, A.V. (1985) *Paid to Care. The Limits of Professionalism in Pastoral Care*. SPCK, London.

James, N. (1989) Emotional labour, skills and work in the social regulation of feeling. *The Sociological Review*, 37 (1), 15–42.

Jones, P.S. and Meleis, A.I. (1993) Health is empowerment. *Advances in Nursing Science*, 15 (3), 1–14.

Kendall, S. (1993) Do health visitors promote client participation? An analysis of the health visitor–client interaction. *Journal of Clinical Nursing*, 2, 103–109.

Kitson, A.L. (1987) A comparative analysis of lay-caring and professional (nursing) caring relationships. *International Journal of Nursing Studies*, 24 (2), 155–165.

Kleinman, A. (1988) *The Illness Narratives: Suffering, Healing and the Human Condition*. Basic Books, New York.

Maben, J., Latter, S., MacLeod Clark, J. and Wilson-Barnett, J. (1993) The organisation of care: its influence on health education practice on acute wards. *Journal of Clinical Nursing*, 2, 355–362.

Malin, N. & Teasedale, K. (1991) Caring versus empowerment: considerations for nursing practice. *Journal of Advanced Nursing*, 16, 657–662.

Melia, K.M. (1987) *Learning and Working. The Occupational Socialisation of Nurses*. Tavistock, London.

Morrison, P. (1991) The caring attitude in nursing practice: a repertory grid study of trained nurses' perceptions. *Nurse Education Today*, 11, 3–12.

Morrison, P. and Bauer, I. (1993) A clinical application of the multiple sorting technique. *International Journal of Nursing Studies*, 30 (6), 511–518.

Nguyen, T.D., Atkinson, C.C. and Stenger, B.L. (1983) Assessment of patient satisfaction: development and refinement of a service evaluation questionnaire. *Evaluation and Program Planning*, 6, 299–314.

Nicholls, K.A. (1993) *Psychological in Physical Illness*. Chapman and Hall, London.

Roberts, S.J. and Khouse, H.J. (1990) Negotiation as a strategy to empower self-care. *Holistic Nursing Practice*, 4 (2), 30–36.

Smith, P. (1992) *The Emotional Labour of Nursing. Its Impact on Interpersonal Relations, Management and the Educational Environment in Nursing*. Macmillan, London.

Strauss, A., Fagerhaugh, S., Suczek, B. and Wiener, C. (1982) The work of hospitalised patients. *Social Science and Medicine*, 16, 977–986.

Strauss, A., Fagerhaugh, S., Suczek, B. and Wiener, C. (1982) Sentimental work in the technologized hospital. *Sociology of Health and Illness*, 4 (3), 254–278.

Chapter 9
Conclusion

Most of us have a vague 'feeling' that things are moving faster. Doctors and executives alike complain that they cannot keep up with the latest developments in their fields. Hardly a meeting or conference takes place today without some ritualistic oratory about 'the challenge of change'. Among many there is an uneasy mood—a suspicion that change is out of control (Toffler, 1970).

Introduction

In this final chapter some of the potential areas of application for the phenomenological approach discussed throughout the book are described. This potential will not be realized overnight. It will take time and effort to evoke changes in individuals and in organizations. It will require personal changes of attitude and behaviour as well as changes in the way care is managed. The effort to change will not be wasted. Patients will benefit greatly from changes in your professional practice. Nurses who work at using this perspective will receive greater job satisfaction from knowing that they have developed their skills in understanding patients and through using that understanding to guide their work as a nurse.

Phenomenological psychology as an approach to understanding patients

The phenomenological approach advocated here is sophisticated enough to enable practitioners to take account of the lived world that other people experience. If nurses and other healthcare workers really want to reduce the gap between theory and practice (rhetoric versus reality), then the capacity to *understand* the views of others is an essential requirement for any such undertaking. The approach advocated here provides a framework for developing truly caring relationships. Pellegrino (1982) reminded us that:

> The fact of illness afflicts our humanity and diminishes it and renders us less able to function as moral agents and as human persons. Illness wounds, diminishes, and compromises our very humanity and places us in a uniquely vulnerable situation in relation to the professed healer. The relationship of healing is inherently one of inequality, vulnerability. The obligations of those who profess to heal directly—the health professionals—and those who provide the conditions requisite for healing transactions—hospitals, teams, or governments— are grounded in the phenomenon of illness as it is experienced by human persons—and this is the philosophical source of professional morality (p. 165).

Taking the patients' viewpoint seriously

In a critical account of psychotherapy, Smail (1991) argued that many conventional approaches to therapy were lacking:

> ... a systematic elaboration of how the distress which therapists encounter in their patients becomes intelligible through being placed within the context which gave rise to it in the first place ... [they] fail to take sufficiently seriously into account the world in which psychological subjects are located (p. 62).

It was suggested that psychologists and therapists needed to adopt a broader environmental perspective in which the important influences on the world of the client in therapy was acknowledged. A similar argument could be put for nurses and other professional helping groups. The approach advocated by Smail is similar to the lifeworld understanding that has been developed in the present text. The depth of insight gained when this approach is used is clearly demonstrated in the previous chapters of the book. The sensitive comprehension gleaned through this method may be used to positively transform the quality of care experienced by patients and their families at a time of illness and personal distress. Both nurses and therapists can employ this perspective provided that appropriate teaching and training are given. One of the difficulties of achieving this goal is the lack of suitable training materials. Another obstacle is the rather complex and obscure language that the reader meets with for the first time.

Another significant element has been the scarcity of readable research reports that convey directly the potential of this approach for practice disciplines such as nursing, psychology and other caring professions. While several starting points exist (Keen, 1975; Kleinman, 1988; Spinelli, 1989), more detailed and clearly written studies are needed. The present account may serve as a helpful introduction to practitioners, educators and researchers. It should help to provide a useful and more tangible means of overcoming some of the barriers to application for the novice, but it is only an introduction.

The approach could also lead to better informed policies that are guided by the perspectives of both patient and professional carer. If we are clear about what patients want and how they react, then we are in a much stronger position to provide this. If we continue to act according to our (professional) perspective, and act according to how we believe patients think and feel, then we are unlikely to meet the patients' expectations and needs successfully. An approach that takes the 'consumers' view seriously needs to take account of the patients' perspective. Such an approach may have direct implications for what we do as practitioners.

Putting the approach to work

At the beginning of this book you read about the phenomenological approach to psychological research and later you read
about some of the details derived from interviews with patients
that were guided by this approach. You now have to evaluate
the potential uses for such an approach in nursing or in other
fields of healthcare. After considering this question myself for
some time I think that the areas mentioned below will lead to
applications that are viable and potentially very useful. All
efforts to use the approach will take time, so the 'pace' of any
innovations needs to be right and an attitude of patience and
commitment will be needed always. The approach could be
used successfully in nursing research, education and practice.
In addition, although the whole tone of the book has a
deliberate 'nursing' perspective, other healthcare workers
could use the approach equally well. The following four main
areas of possible application include:

Nurse education and nursing practice

The approach could help nurses to be clearer about how they
want the profession to develop. As part of the educational
process, students undergo 'professional socialization' (Davis,
1975; Melia, 1987; Simpson, 1979) during which they acquire
shared values, attitudes and behaviours across the organization.
Professional socialization has a critical part to play in the
development of professional individuals who care about people. This process also leads to the establishment of 'caring
institutions'.

However, it should not be assumed that the system of
education and the world of work in which professional caring
is administered always share the same goals. Clearly they do
not (Ashworth and Morrison, 1989; Melia, 1987). Using the
example of professional socialization in medical students to

support this view, Kleinman (1988) argued that professional socialization produced doctors that he referred to as 'disabled' healers:

> Professional training, in principle then, should make it feasible for practitioners to deliver care that is both technically competent and humane whether or not they are personally motivated toward a particular patient or work under threatening conditions. Certain aspects of professional training seem to disable practitioners. The professional mask may protect the individual practitioner from feelings of being overwhelmed by patients' demands; but it also may cut him off from the human experience of illness (p. 225).

A very similar training pattern can be seen in the nursing profession (Menzies, 1970). In truth very little attention is paid to the human component of nursing work. In these days of 'market forces' philosophy, it would appear that expensive training serves to produce a system that is more concerned with the process and outcomes of professional care rather than the content (other vulnerable and ill human beings). The emphasis on management by qualified nurses and the need to become more management orientated to secure promotion are clear examples of what happens in practice.

One possible solution might be to appoint ward managers (nurses with special management aptitude and training) and let the trained nurses 'nurse' patients directly. If we do not clarify how we want to develop we leave ourselves open to being forced into a role with less and less patient contact. This suggests another possibility for dealing with the above problem. To a manager of services it may make more economic sense to employ more untrained or less well-trained people to provide the 'caring' or 'human' contact with patients and acknowledge that the trained nurses (the procedural or technical experts) do not really need to get involved in this aspect of nursing people. This latter scenario may be the cost of achieving higher 'professional' status as nurses—the trained nurses become managers with no direct patient contact.

If the implicit desire within the profession is to 'care for people', which means having contact with people who happen to be ill, and this desire is built upon a natural helping attitude that many learners bring with them to the job, then this attitude needs to be fostered during a period of socialization. For this to happen, learners need good role models and a supportive learning environment (Pratt, 1980). It has been suggested that:

> ... caring is not being learned, because, in general, it is not being either taught or demonstrated with sufficient purpose (Pratt, 1980, p. 52).

It is the responsibility of practitioners, as well as the teaching, administrative and policy-making staff, to ensure these requirements are not overlooked *if* we really want to emphasize the psychological side of the nursing role.

It also remains to be seen if it is possible to get students and practising nurses to begin to think about their patients from a phenomenological perspective. Obviously some nurses already do, but not as a matter of course. The system does not promote such an outlook; it moulds even the most caring and innovative individuals into organizational functionaries. Training workshops and exercises could be designed and developed. I have myself developed with a colleague some of my ideas into a student text and teaching manual to try and promote such a perspective in educational institutions (Morrison and Burnard, 1991a, b). In these texts we have adopted Kelly's personal construct theory and repertory grid technique to promote the phenomenological perspective along with Heron's Six Category Intervention Analysis (Heron, 1989) and The Counsellor Attitude Scale (Nelson-Jones and Patterson, 1975).

Keen (1975) claimed that the personal construct theory approach along with the repertory grid technique was one of the methods that could be used fruitfully by phenomenological psychologists. He wrote:

> The whole point of Kelly's exercise is finally to make clear
> that there are alternative ways to perceive people—indeed to
> construe the world and thus to structure that space among
> people within which we live and move everyday ... We have
> here almost a routine that can teach the phenomenological-
> reduction and imaginative-variation techniques for seeing
> more clearly what and how and why we see as we do (Keen,
> 1975, p. 66).

More techniques and training packages need to be developed
and these should be even more qualitative. In addition, new
teaching developments must help students to get to grips with
important methodological issues and explore the range of
applications in 'real world' settings. The packages we have
developed represent a first step, but much more work needs to
be done. This book is a further step in this direction. If teachers
want students to really understand patients, then we must teach
them how to do this in a professional context.

Nursing research

Several helpful papers exist that convey the essential principles
of the phenomenological method used here, but few seem to be
written in a straightforward manner and are often in rather
inaccessible journals. Good methodological papers are often
not directly applicable to the field of nursing or psychological
healthcare research. All these issues are likely to inhibit
potential users from taking up this approach. A detailed
description of the method used to analyse the interview data
has been reported elsewhere (Morrison, 1991, 1992). In addition, the detailed description of the patients' experiences
outlined here should prove to be helpful to others attempting to
get to grips with this approach and give clues as to the type and
quality of understanding that may be achieved in a research
study using this approach.

Those hoping to use the approach in research studies will (I hope) find this book informative, but they will quickly identify a need to explore some of the methodological principles in greater depth and breadth before undertaking a study grounded in this approach. Identifying a suitable and experienced research supervisor will be an essential first step.

Applications for other professional carers

Although this book is written with nursing students and practitioners in mind, clearly many of the issues discussed here, while having direct relevance to the work of the nurse, are relevant for other healthcare workers. Clinical psychologists, counsellors, therapists, social workers, occupational therapists and physiotherapists all have contact with 'people as patients'. Some of these are community based while others work mainly in institutional settings.

These professional groups share some common factors in their roles as professional helpers: they need to *understand* patients and they are *paid to care* for patients. The approach outlined here could help these professionals to work more effectively and to benefit themselves and their patients. Informal carers such as volunteers, advice and information agencies, or relatives who care for the chronically ill and disabled in their own homes could also benefit from learning about the approach and putting it into practice. However, we need to focus on the professional groups first.

Research on particular groups

This approach has particular significance for studying particular groups of clients or informants. Research studies could be performed with specific groups of staff and patients. Toombs (1992), for example, highlighted differences in the perspectives of physicians and patients. A detailed account of the sort of caring experienced by AIDS patients, cancer patients, the chronically sick and disabled, the mentally ill and the mentally disabled, for example, could prove to be particularly useful. In addition, studies in these and similar areas could play an important role in the development of policies and practices that are genuinely caring and *reflect a concern for both carer and client*.

Moreover, these types of studies could help to develop theory that really does reflect everyday practice issues for professional carers. The practitioners of nursing should be particularly vigilant to ensure that the concerns of the clients or patients we claim to care for are an integral part of the care they receive. We need to focus more on patients. This emphasis may lead to more collaborative studies with other professional helping groups such as doctors, psychologists, occupational therapists and physiotherapists.

What can be done to improve the situation

Nurses can do several things to help change the impact of the hospital environment on patients. Reading this book is a good starting point, but there is still a need to read more about the approach used in this book and really try to understand the essential principles of the phenomenological method described in Chapter 2. Try to imagine a style of nursing that is based on the principles discussed here and consider how different nursing assessments might be if professional assessments and judgements about patients were made along these lines. Keep thinking about this and focus on the positive outcomes that could follow. If you can imagine bringing about important changes in your own nursing practice, it is also possible to bring about those changes in reality.

Nurses generally work in teams and the approach described here has potential for individuals and for nurses who work as part of a team. Bringing about changes in settled teams poses extra problems and requires some additional thought, but it is nevertheless possible to elicit change in colleagues. West (1989) identified and described four crucial factors that are important in eliciting change in organizations and professional teams. These were:

- Having a shared vision of what is important—this is the vision that the staff group have and value. An example may be a desire to get patients to become more responsible and independent. These are best developed within the staff group because those handed down from on high often have little impact because their originators are not familiar enough with the day-to-day work of the organization. The goals must be achievable. If they are not then people will become demotivated.
- Participative safety—this means that people must *participate* in developments. Higher levels of participation lead to greater innovations. This does not mean that everybody in the work group should agree on every issue, but everyone should feel secure enough to discuss and debate the pros and cons of particular strategies. The important thing is for people to feel confident to take part in discussions about developments. Having regular social events and promoting a climate of openness and honesty are most helpful too.
- Commitment to excellent work—staff need to be highly motivated to achieving excellence in their work. A wide range of strategies to achieve this is evident and indeed tolerated by co-workers committed to innovations. There may be controversy and heated debate and this is absolutely necessary to enable minority views (such as those of students) to be expressed. It has been shown that minority opinions can promote innovations.
- Supportive structure for innovation—if change and innovations are to occur, they need to be supported. Verbal

support for new ideas is also needed, but concrete support with time and resources are essential if developments are to take place. People need time to think and talk amongst each other to develop plans for implementing these ideas. They may need space and some financial support.

Much can be achieved at ward level if people are committed to building a ward culture that incorporates these four criteria. If these characteristics are present, then you are much more likely to elicit change and innovation in your work setting. Moreover, the *quantity* and the *quality* of group innovation is much higher when these characteristics are in evidence (West, 1989).

A final note

I hope that you have enjoyed reading this book and, what is more important, that I have been successful in making you *think* more about your work. We have a long way to go to match our stated aim of being a 'caring' profession. I believe that the approach described here provides a template for achieving that goal, but it will take time and patience and a great deal of hard work.

Further reading

Beail, N. (1985) *Repertory Grid Technique and Personal Constructs. Applications in Clinical and Educational Settings*. Croom Helm, London.

Fisher, W. (1970) The faces of anxiety. *Journal of Phenomenological Psychology*, 1, 21–50.

Georgiades, N.J. and Phillimore, L. (1975) The myth of the hero-innovator and alternative strategies for organisational change. In: C.C. Kiernan and P. Woodford (eds) *Behaviour*

Modification with the Severely Retarded. Associated Scientific Publishers, Amsterdam, pp. 313–319.

Hall, J. (1990) Towards a psychology of caring. *British Journal of Clinical Psychology*, 29, 129–144.

Heider, F. (1958) *The Psychology of Interpersonal Relations.* Wiley, New York.

Huczynski, A. and Buchanan, D. (1991) *Organisational Behaviour.* 2nd edn. Prentice Hall, London.

Kelly, G.A. (1955) *The Psychology of Personal Constructs,* vols 1, 2. Norton, New York.

McIver, S. (1993) *Obtaining The Views of Users of Health Services About Quality of Information.* King's Fund Centre, London.

Morrison, P. and Burnard, P. (1991a) *Caring and Communicating. The Interpersonal Relationship in Nursing.* Macmillan, Basingstoke.

Morrison, P. and Burnard, P. (1991b) *Caring and Communicating. Facilitators Manual.* Macmillan, Basingstoke.

Nemeth, C.J. and Wachtler, J. (1983) Creative problem solving as a result of majority vs minority influence. *European Journal of Social Psychology*, 13, 45–55.

Towell, D. & Dartington, T. (1976) Encouraging innovations in hospital care. *Journal of Advanced Nursing*, 4, 403–413.

Towell, D. & Harries, C. (1979) *Innovations in Patient Care.* Croom Helm, London.

West, M. (1989) Visions and team innovation. *Changes*, 7, 115–122.

West, M.A. and Farr, J.L. (1989) Innovation at work: psychological perspectives. *Social Behaviour*, 4, 15–30.

References

Abraham, C. and Shanley, E. (1992) *Social Psychology for Nurses. Understanding Interaction in Health Care*. Edward Arnold, London.

Abramson, L.Y. and Martin, D.J. (1981) Depression and the causal inference process. In: J.M. Harvey, W. Ickes and R.F. Kidd (eds) *New Directions in Attribution Research*. Vol. 3. Erlbaum, Hillsdale, New Jersey.

Abramson, L.Y., Seligman, M.E.P. and Teasdale, J.D. (1978) Learned helplessness in humans: critique and reformulation. *Journal of Abnormal Psychology*, 87, 49–74.

Ashworth, P. and Morrison, P. (1989) Some ambiguities of the students' role in undergraduate nurse training. *Journal of Advanced Nursing*, 14, 1009–1015.

Ashworth, P., Longmate, A. and Morrison, P. (1992) Patient participation: its meaning and significance in the context of caring. *Journal of Advanced Nursing*, 17, 1430–1439.

Atkinson, R.L., Atkinson, R.C., Smith, E.E. and Bem, D.J. (1990) *Introduction to Psychology*, 10th edn. Harcourt Brace Jovanovich, London.

Audit Commission (1993) *What Seems to be the Matter: Communication Between Hospitals and Patients*. HMSO, London.

Baron, R.A and Byrne, D. (1987) *Social Psychology. Understanding Human Interaction*. Allyn and Bacon, Boston.

Bartjes, A. (1991) Phenomenology in clinical practice. In: G. Gray and M. Pratt (eds) *Towards a Discipline of Nursing*. Churchill Livingstone, Melbourne, pp. 247–264.

Benner, P. (1984) *From Novice to Expert. Excellence and*

Power in Clinical Nursing Practice. Addison-Wesley, London.

Benner, P. and Wrubel, J. (1989) *The Primacy of Caring: Stress and Coping in Health and Illness.* Addison-Wesley, Menlo Park, California.

Bernstein, R. (1983) *Beyond Objectivism and Relativism.* University of Pennsylvania Press, Philadelphia.

Boud, D. (1985) Problem-based learning in perspective. In D. Boud (ed.) *Problem Based Learning in Education for the Professions.* Higher Education Research and Development Society of Australasia, Sydney, pp. 13–18.

Broome, A.K. (ed.) (1989) *Health Psychology. Processes and Applications.* Chapman and Hall, London.

Buber, M. (1958) *I and Thou*, 2nd edn. T&T Clark, Edinburgh.

Buber, M. (1966) In: M. Friedman (ed.) *The Knowledge of Man: A Philosophy of the Interhuman.* (Translated by R.G. Smith.) Harper and Row, New York.

Burnard, P. (1989) *Counselling Skills for Health Professionals.* Chapman and Hall, London.

Campbell, A.V. (1985) *Paid to Care. The Limits of Professionalism in Pastoral Care.* SPCK, London.

Cassee, E.T.H. (1975) Therapeutic behaviour, hospital culture and communication. In: C. Cox and A. Mead (eds) *A Sociology of Medical Practice.* Collier-Macmillan, London, pp. 224–234.

Chapman, C.M. (1983) The paradox of nursing. *Journal of Advanced Nursing*, 8, 269–272.

Cooper, I.S. (1976) *Living with Chronic Neurologic Disease.* Norton, New York.

Cormack, D. (1976) *Psychiatric Nursing Observed. A Descriptive Study of the Work of the Charge Nurse in Acute Admission Wards of Psychiatric Hospitals.* RCN, London.

Coser, R.L. (1962) *Life in the Ward.* Michigan State University, Michigan.

Cowen, E.L. (1982) Help where you find it. Four informal helping groups. *American Psychologist*, 37 (4), 385–395.

Davis, F. (1975) Professional socialisation as subjective experience: the process of doctrinal conversion among student nurses. In: C. Cox and A. Mead (eds) *A Sociology of Medical Practice*. Collier-Macmillan, London, pp. 116–131.

Davis, H. and Fallowfield, L. (eds) (1991) *Counselling and Communication in Health Care*. Wiley, Chichester.

Devine, E.C. and Cook, T.D. (1983) A meta-analytical analysis of effects of psycho-educational interventions on length of post surgical hospital stay. *Nursing Research*, 32 (5), 267–274.

Drew, N. (1986) Exclusion and confirmation: a phenomenology of patients' experiences of caregivers. *Image: Journal of Nursing Scholarship*, 18 (2), 39–43.

Dunlop, M.J. (1986) Is a science of caring possible? *Journal of Advanced Nursing*, 11, 661–670.

Evers, H.K. (1986) Care of the elderly sick in the UK. In: S.J. Redfern (ed.) *Nursing Elderly People*. Churchill Livingstone, Edinburgh, pp. 293–310.

Fallowfield, L. (1991) *Breast Cancer*. Tavistock/Routledge, London.

Ferguson, B.F. (1979) Preparing young children for hospitalisation. *Pediatrics*, 64, 656–664.

Friedman, M. (1985) Healing through meeting and the problem of mutuality. *Journal of Humanistic Psychology*, 25 (1), 7–40.

Gadow, S. (1980) Existential advocacy: philosophical foundation of nursing. In: S.F. Spicker and S. Gadow (eds) *Nursing: Images and Ideals: Opening Dialogue with the Humanities*. Springer, New York, pp. 79–101.

Giorgi, A. (1970) *Psychology as a Human Science: a Phenomenologically Based Approach*. Harper and Row, New York.

Giorgi, A., Fisher, W.F. and Von Eckartsberg, R. (eds) (1971) *Duquesne Studies in Phenomenological Psychology*, vol. I. Duquesne University Press, Pittsburgh.

Gleitman, H. (1992) *Basic Psychology*, 3rd edn. Norton, London.

Goffman, E. (1956) The nature of deference and demeanour. *American Anthropologist*, 58 (3), 473–502.

Goffman, E. (1968) *Asylums: Essays on the Social Situation of Mental Patients and Other Inmates*. Penguin, Harmondsworth.

Goodman, C. (1986) Research on the informal carer: a selected literature review. *Journal of Advanced Nursing*, 11, 705–712.

Greenberg, M.S. and Westcott, D.R. (1982) Indebtedness as a mediator of reactions to aid. In: J.D. Fisher, A. Nadler and B.M. DePaulo (eds) *New Directions in Helping: Recipient Reactions to Aid*, vol. 1. Academic Press, New York, pp. 85–112.

Guggenbühl-Craig, A. (1971) *Power in the Helping Professions*. Spring, University of Dallas, Irving, Texas.

Gullickson, C. (1993) My death nearing its future: a Heideggerian hermeneutical analysis of the lived experience of persons with chronic illness. *Journal of Advanced Nursing*, 18, 1386–1392.

Heidegger, M. (1962) *Being and Time*. (Translated by J. Macquarrie and E. Robinson). Basil Blackwell, Oxford.

Heider, F. (1958) *The Psychology of Interpersonal Relations*. Wiley, New York.

Heron, J. (1989) *Six Category Intervention Analysis*, 3rd edn. Croom Helm, London.

Hirschfeld, M. (1983) Home care versus institutionalization: family caregiving and senile brain disease. *International Journal of Nursing Studies*, 20 (1), 23–32.

Holmes, C.A. (1990) Alternatives to natural science foundations for nursing. *International Journal of Nursing Studies*, 27 (3), 187–198.

Hugman, R. (1991) *Power in Caring Professions*. Macmillan, London.

Husserl, E. (1972) *Ideas: General Introduction to Pure Phenomenology*. (Translations by W.R. Boyce.) Collier, New York.

Hycner, R.H. (1985) Some guidelines for the phenomenological analysis of interview data. *Human Studies*, 8, 279–303.

Illich, I. (1975) *Medical Nemesis: The Expropriation of Health*. Calder and Boyars, London.

Jeffrey, R. (1979) Normal rubbish: deviant patients in casualty departments. *Sociology of Health and Illness*, 1 (1), 90–107.

Jourard, S. (1964) *The Transparent Self*. Van Nostrand, Princeton, New Jersey.

Keen, E. (1975) *A Primer in Phenomenological Psychology*. Holt, Rinehart and Winston, New York. (Reprinted in 1982 by University Press of America, Lanham.)

Kelly, G.A. (1955) *The Psychology of Personal Constructs*. vols 1, 2. Norton, New York.

Kelly, G.A. (1963) *A Theory of Personality*. Norton, London.

Kelly, M.P. and May, P. (1982) Good and bad patients: a review of the literature and a theoretical critique. *Journal of Advanced Nursing*, 7, 147–156.

Kent, G. and Dalgleish, M. (1986) *Psychology and Medical Care*. 2nd edn. Baillière Tindall, London.

Kestenbaum, V. (ed.) (1982a) *The Humanity of the Ill: Phenomenological Perspectives*. University of Tennessee Press, Knoxville.

Kestenbaum, V. (1982b) Introduction: the experience of illness. In: V. Kestenbaum (ed.) *The Humanity of the Ill: Phenomenological Perspectives*. University of Tennessee Press, Knoxville, pp. 3–38.

Kitson, A.L. (1987a) Raising standards of clinical practice—

the fundamental issue of effective nursing practice. *Journal of Advanced Nursing*, 12, 321–329.

Kitson, A.L. (1987b) A comparative analysis of lay-caring and professional (nursing) caring relationships. *International Journal of Nursing Studies*, 24 (2), 155–165.

Kleinman, A. (1988) *The Illness Narratives: Suffering, Healing and the Human Condition*. Basic Books, New York.

Knight, M. and Field, D. (1981) Silent conspiracy: coping with dying cancer patients on acute surgical wards. *Journal of Advanced Nursing*, 6, 221–229.

Kvale, S. (1983) The qualitative research interview: a phenomenological and hermeneutical mode of understanding. *Journal of Phenomenological Psychology*, 14 (2), 171–196.

Lefcourt, H.M. (1973) The function of the illusions of control and freedom. *American Psychologist*, 28, 417–425.

Leigh, H. and Reiser, M.E. (1980) *The Patient. Biological, Psychological, and Social Dimensions of Medical Practice*. Plenum, New York.

Lenrow, P. (1978) Dilemmas of professional helping: continuities and discontinuities with folk helping roles. In: L. Wispe (ed.) *Altruism, Sympathy, and Helping: Psychological and Sociological Principles*. Academic Press, New York, pp. 263–290.

Ley, P. (1988) *Communicating with Patients: Improving Communication, Satisfaction and Compliance*. Chapman and Hall, London.

Ley, P. (1989) Improving patients' understanding, recall, satisfaction and compliance. In: A.K. Broome (ed.) *Health Psychology. Processes and Applications*. Chapman and Hall, London.

Lofland, J. and Lofland, L.H. (1984) *Analysing Social Settings. A Guide to Qualitative Observation and Analysis*, 2nd edn. Wadsworth, Belmont, California.

Lorber, J. (1975) Good patients and problem patients: conformity and deviance in a general hospital. *Journal of Health and Social Behaviour*, 16 (2), 213–225.

Macquarrie, J. (1973) *Existentialism: An Introduction, Guide and Assessment*. Penguin, Harmondsworth.

May, C. (1990) Research on nurse–patient relationships: problems of theory, problems of practice. *Journal of Advanced Nursing*, 15, 307–315.

May, D. and Kelly, M.P. (1982) Chancers pests and pour wee souls: problems of legitimation in psychiatric illness. *Sociology of Health and Illness*, 4 (3), 279–301.

Melia, K.M. (1987) *Learning and Working. The Occupational Socialization of Nurses*. Tavistock, London.

Menzies, I.E.P. (1970) *The Functioning of Social Systems as a Defence Against Anxiety*. Centre for Applied Social Research, Tavistock Institute of Human Relations, London.

Miller, A. (1985) Nurse/patient dependency—is it iatrogenic. *Journal of Advanced Nursing*, 10, 63–69.

Miller, J.F. (1992) *Coping with Chronic Illness. Overcoming Powerlessness*. F.A. Davis, Philadelphia.

Morgan, M. (1991) Hospitals and patients. In: G. Scrambler (ed.) *Sociology as Applied to Medicine*, 3rd edn. Baillière Tindall, London.

Morrison, P. (1991) *The Meaning of Caring Interpersonal Relationships in Nursing*. PhD thesis, Sheffield Hallam University, Sheffield.

Morrison, P. (1992) *Professional Caring in Practice. A Psychological Analysis*. Avebury, Aldershot.

Morrison, P. and Bauer, I. (1993) A clinical application of the multiple sorting technique. *International Journal of Nursing Studies*, 30 (6), 511–518.

Morrison, P. and Burnard, P. (1991a) *Caring and Communicating. The Interpersonal Relationship in Nursing*. Macmillan, Basingstoke.

Morrison, P. and Burnard, P. (1991b) *Caring and Communicating. Facilitators Manual*. Macmillan, Basingstoke.

Morse J. (ed.) (1989) *Qualitative Nursing Research: A Contemporary Dialogue*. Aspen, Rockville, Maryland.

Morse, J.M. (1991) Negotiating commitment and involvement in the nurse–patient relationship. *Journal of Advanced Nursing*, 16, 455–468.

Nehring, V. and Geach, B. (1973) Patients' evaluation of their care: why they don't complain. *Nursing Outlook*, 21 (5), 317–321.

Nelson-Jones, R. and Patterson, C.H. (1975) Measuring the client-centres attitudes. *British Journal of Guidance and Counselling*, 3 (2), 228–236.

Neyle, D. and West, S. (1991) In support of a scientific method. In: G. Gray and R. Pratt (eds) *Towards a Discipline of Nursing*. Churchill Livingstone, Melbourne, pp. 265–284.

Nichols, K.A. (1993) *Psychological Care in Physical Illness*. Chapman and Hall, London.

Nordholm, L.A. (1980) Beautiful patients are good patients: evidence for the physical attractiveness stereotype in first impressions of patients. *Social Science and Medicine*, 14A, 81–83.

Olesen, V.L. and Whittaker, E.W. (1968) *The Silent Dialogue: A Study in the Social Psychology of Professional Socialisation*. Jossey-Bass, San Francisco.

Omery, A. (1983) Phenomenology: a method for nursing research. *Advances in Nursing Science*, 5 (2), 49–63.

Orne, M.T. (1962) On the social psychology of the psychological experiment: with particular reference to demand characteristics and their implications. *American Psychologist*, 17, 776–783.

Parsons, T. (1951) *The Social System*. Routledge and Kegan Paul, London.

Paterson, J.G. and Zderad, L.T. (1988) *Humanistic Nursing*. National League for Nursing, New York. (Originally published in 1976.)

Pellegrino, E.D. (1982) Being ill and being healed; some reflections on the grounding of medical morality. In: V. Kestenbaum (ed.) *The Humanity of the Ill: Phenomenological Perspectives*. University of Tennessee Press, Knoxville, pp. 157–166.

Pendleton, D.A. and Bochner, S. (1980) The communication of medical information in general practice consultations as a function of patients' social class. *Social Science and Medicine*, 14A, 669–673.

Pennington, D.C. (1986) *Essential Social Psychology*. Edward Arnold, London.

Pratt, R. (1980) A time to every purpose … *The Australian Nurses' Journal*, 10 (3), 50–53, 56.

Rempusheski, V.F., Chamberlain, S.L., Picard, H.B., Ruzanski, J. and Collier, M. (1988) Expected and received care: patient perceptions. *Nursing Administration Quarterly*, 12 (3), 42–50.

Robinson, J., Stilwell, J., Hawley, C. and Hempstead, N. (1989) *The Role of the Support Worker in the Ward Health Care Team*. Nursing Policy Studies Centre and Health Service Research Unit, University of Warwick.

Robinson, L. (1968) *Psychological Aspects of the Care of Hospitalised Patients*. F.A. Davis, Philadelphia.

Rogers, A., Pilgrim, D. and Lacy, R. (1993) *Experiencing Psychiatry. Users' Views of Services*. Macmillan, Basingstoke.

Rogers, C.R. (1967) *On Becoming a Person: a Therapist's View of Psychotherapy*. Constable, London.

Rogers, W.S. (1991) *Explaining Health and Illness. An Exploration of Diversity*. Harvester Wheatsheaf, London.

Sacks, O. (1985) *The Man who Mistook His Wife for a Hat*. Picador, London.

Schulz, R. and Aderman, D. (1974) Effect of residential change on the temporal distance to death of terminal cancer patients. *Omega: Journal of Death and Dying*, 2, 157–162.

Schutz, A. (1962) *Collected Papers 1: The Problem of Social Reality*. Martinus Nijhoff, The Hague.

Seligman, M.E.P. (1992) *Helplessness: On Depression, Development and Death*. Freeman, San Francisco.

Seligman, M.E.P., Abramson, L.Y., Semmel, A. and Von Baeyer, C. (1979) Depressive attributional style. *Journal of Abnormal Psychology*, 88, 242–247.

Simpson, I.H. (1979) *From Student to Nurse: A Longitudinal Study of Socialisation*. Cambridge University Press, Cambridge.

Skipper, J.K. and Leonard, R. (1968) Children, stress and hospitalisation: a field experiment. *Journal of Health and Social Behaviour*, 9, 275–287.

Skipper, J.K., Tagliacozzo, D. and Mauksch, H. (1964) Some possible consequences of limited communication between patients and hospital functionaries. *Journal of Health and Human Behavior*, 5, 34–39.

Smail, D. (1991) Towards a radical environmentalist psychology of help. *The Psychologist*, 2, 61–65.

Smith, P. (1992) *The Emotional Labour of Nursing. Its Impact on Interpersonal Relations, Management and the Educational Environment in Nursing*. Macmillan, London.

Spiegelberg, H. (1982) *The Phenomenological Movement: A Historical Introduction*. 3rd edn. Martinus Nijhoff, The Hague.

Spinelli, E. (1989) *The Interpreted World: An Introduction to Phenomenological Psychology*. Sage, London.

Stevenson, L. (1987) *Seven Theories of Human Nature*. 2nd edn. Oxford University Press, Oxford.

Stockwell, F. (1972) *The Unpopular Patient*. RCN, London.

Strauss, A., Fagerhaugh, S., Suczek, B. and Wiener, C. (1982a) The work of hospitalised patients. *Social Science and Medicine*, 16, 977–986.

Strauss, A., Fagerhaugh, S., Suczek, B. and Wiener, C. (1982b)

Sentimental work in the technologized hospital. *Sociology of Health and Illness*, 4 (3), 254–278.

Swanson-Kauffman, K. and Schonwald, E. (1988) Phenomenology. In: B. Sarter (ed.) *Paths to Knowledge: Innovative Research Methods for Nursing*. National League for Nursing, New York, pp. 97–105.

Taylor, S. (1979) Hospital patient behavior: reactance, helplessness, or control. *Journal of Social Issues*, 35 (1), 156–184.

Taylor, S.J. and Bogdan, R. (1984) *Introduction to Qualitative Research Methods. The Search for Meanings*, 2nd edn. Wiley, New York.

Toffler, A. (1970) *Future Shock*. Pan Books, London.

Toombs, S.K. (1992) *The Meaning of Illness. A Phenomenological Account of the Different Perspectives of Physician and Patient*. Kluwer, London.

Towell, D. (1975) *Understanding Psychiatric Nursing: A Sociological Study of Modern Psychiatric Nursing Practice*. RCN, London.

Valle, R.S., King, M. and Halling, S. (1989) An introduction to existential-phenomenological thought in psychology. In: R.S. Valle and S. Halling (eds) *Existential-Phenomenological Perspectives in Psychology: Exploring the Breadth of Human Experience*. Plenum, New York, pp. 3–16.

Van den Berg, J.H. (1972a) *A Different Existence: Principles of Phenomenological Psychopathology*. Duquesne University Press, Pittsburgh, PA.

Van den Berg, J.H. (1972b) *The Psychology of the Sickbed*. Humanities Press, New York.

Van Manen, M. (1990) *Researching Lived Experience: Human Science for an Action Sensitive Pedagogy*. The Althouse Press, Ontario.

Wallston, B.S. and Wallston, K.A. (1978) Locus of control and health: a review of the literature. *Health Education Monographs*, 6, 107–111.

Waterworth, S. and Luker, K. (1990) Reluctant collaborators: Do patients want to be involved in decisions concerning care? *Journal of Advanced Nursing* 15, 971–976.

Watson, J. (1979) *Nursing: The Philosophy and Science of Caring*. Little Brown, Boston.

Watson, J. (1985) *Nursing: Human Science and Human Care: A Theory of Nursing*. Appleton-Century-Crofts, New York.

Weiner, B. (1980) A cognitive (attribution)–emotion–action model of motivated behaviour: an analysis of judgements of help-giving. *Journal of Personality and Social Psychology*, 39 (2), 186–200.

West, M. (1989) Visions and team innovation. *Changes*, 7, 115–122.

Wilkes, L. (1991) Phenomenology: a window to the nursing world. In: G. Gray and M. Pratt (eds) *Towards a Discipline of Nursing*. Churchill Livingstone, Melbourne, pp. 229–246

Index